Praise for *A Pound of Hope*

"I have learned my greatest lessons from my patients; and this book, *A Pound of Hope*, is no exception to that. As a practicing pediatrician for 28 years, it is gratifying to witness and be a part of the advances in health care delivery to extremely premature infants. While this is the story of a well prepared young couple making all the decisions to aid in the success of their children's development and overall health, it is also a cautionary tale of the financial burden that may accompany it. I believe a system could be employed to cover catastrophic events through private insurance pools, just as the government covers certificates of deposit. Our medical care is the best in the world, but it should not bankrupt those who contribute to its cost."

David M. Christopher, MD

"*A Pound of Hope* tells it how it is, so don't expect a sugar coating. This is the moving account of medical procedures you can't bear to watch, and urgent life-altering decisions made in the midst of crisis after crisis. It's a story that changes your perception of the world forever—you'll find yourself acutely aware of the fragility of life, and how poignant every day is that we have with our loved ones."

Shawna Karuna-karan
Mother of a preemie

"Jennifer's journal is filled with love, wisdom and ferocious hope. You will be *undone* by the courage of this family and the medical team that navigates decisions; willing the twins to live and move back from death's edge night after night. *A Pound of Hope* is a wonderful story of love, family and faith. It teaches us simple lessons of how we can help and support friends and neighbors in need."

Patty Warner Kerston, Retired Executive, SAFECO

Praise for *A Pound of Hope*

"As a nurse in the NICU, I found this journal of premature twins remarkably honest in the telling. Nothing is held back. *A Pound of Hope* is a must read for the medical team as it gives us a glimpse into the tender, broken heart of parents so we can be of better support to them in their time of need."

Jeanne Peterson, RN, Neonatal Intensive Care Unit

"*A Pound of Hope* is an incredible story... it lays bare what families deal with when they have a critically ill child. Our medical community can save many of these tiny premature babies—and now we can read the candid perspective on the raw emotional and crushing financial roller coaster that comes with these medical miracles."

Jill Dombey, RN, Neonatal Intensive Care Unit

"One mother's heart-wrenching journey is portrayed in *A Pound of Hope* as she navigates the healthcare system while her critically ill twins struggle for life against all odds. Tones of hope and inspiration echo through their miraculous story of survival, as the book exposes disheartening injustices in healthcare access, financing, and delivery."

Lisa Burke, RN, Pediatric Oncology
Mother of premature twins

"I know firsthand the truth of *A Pound of Hope*. It gives voice to NICU parents and speaks loud and clear on the gaps in medical social services. The real-life examples will tug at your heart, and will help to foster change in social work practice. It's a wakeup call for all of us in medical social services to step up to the challenge.

Luckisha S. Phillips, Medical Social Worker
Mother of a preemie

A Pound of Hope

Second Edition

Michele Munro Kemper
Jennifer Kemper Sinconis

PostScript Publications
Issaquah, WA 98027
USA

Printed and bound in the United States of America

Second Edition 2012 – with added chapters
   Fast Forward: One to Five
   Research for Prevention of Preterm Birth
   Discussion Questions

First Edition 2010

Cover photo by Anthony Saffery

ISBN 978-0615354033

You may contact the authors at: apoundofhope@me.com

Available in paperback or e-book from your favorite bookseller.

For Lou and Eric

Note to Readers

This is a true story—but like all memoirs, the telling is a blend of truth and creative fiction.

The agonizing pace of the medical and financial crises are retold from my personal journals where I faithfully recorded the despair, hope, and joy that came with extremely premature twins. This is the true side of the story, as there was no need to fictionalize to create drama. The life-threatening crises, the daring skill and compassion of the medical team, and the bottomless pit of despair and financial loss—these were all drama enough.

Human beings, not good guys and bad guys, populate this story. I created composite characters, assigned dialogue, and attributed feelings. Names of people and hospitals are changed, and details are jumbled-up for the sake of privacy and discretion—all part of the creative side of re-telling this incredible true story.

TABLE OF CONTENTS

FOREWORD

This book is about Life itself, how the greatest value in any of our lives is to preserve and nurture new life, how we struggle and fight to make Life happen, to keep it going, to fight off despair and darkness and death. *A Pound Of Hope* belongs on the same vibrant, living bookshelf as those stories of parents who swam hundreds of miles in an inner-tube to give their children a decent and safe life, the mothers who handed their babies down to strangers from trains on the way to concentration camps, the fathers in the tsunami who pushed their children to safety as they were swept away themselves. This book defines the value of life, and if it does not make you cry, you have no tear ducts.

I founded the Starlight Children's Foundation in 1982 after helping one seriously ill boy called Sean experience joy shortly before he died. My cousin Emma and I flew Sean 5000 miles from London to Los Angeles, because to him Disneyland was the exact happiness he wanted to experience! And in my apartment where everyone stayed, I saw something else alongside the delight of a very sick little boy having an adventure: I saw his mom, Brenda; enjoy herself too for the first time in years. And I came to understand the unimaginable stress and suffering of all moms and dads when their child is heart-wrenchingly ill. Helping 2.4 million of these families now each year is a delight, a privilege, and an honor.

The emotional and financial wasteland for families that accompanies pediatric illness is not just tragic...some large part of it is unnecessary and man-made. Our society has developed machines and techniques to preserve and extend life against all odds...early life, elderly life, any life at all. But our private and public support systems have not addressed how all this wonderment of medical intervention can possibly be afforded by families stricken with sudden financial burdens that destroy their savings, their future, their very viability. Time and again as Moms and Dads navigate the destruction of their finances, I see not just their financial bankruptcy, but also the dismaying alienation and dismantling of the family unit that comes with never-ending financial stress. Divorce, poverty and the eradication of other opportunities for parents and siblings alike often afflict these good, decent, honorable middle-class families when serious illness amongst them destroys lives and choices.

This has to stop. What is the point of a civilization, a government, medical and insurance systems, the whole infrastructure, if between them they furnish the means to extraordinarily preserve life but make no allowance to pay for it? Even in the new insurance legislation, this category of awfulness gets little attention or remedy. And as the capabilities of medicine thankfully improve exponentially, our leaders so often seem clueless in how these are to be paid for, except by destruction of the very families least able to cope with the stress of their tremendous financial burdens.

The greatest meaning of Life is the procreation and preservation of Life itself; it is the fundamental instinct of our genome and of all living beings. It is what kept our line alive in caves and famines and disasters. It is epic, it is fundamental, and it is who we are as people. In the story of Jen and Justin there is despair and tragedy, but in the end joy and laughter. They won their mortal battle, fought back the darkness and made sure their sons Aidan and Ethan survived and thrived. Their story takes place in a hospital NICU, but it transcends both time and place…it is the story of Life itself.

Peter Samuelson
TV and Film Producer/Executive Producer
Founder, Starlight Children's Foundation
www.starlight.org

PREFACE

Our identical twin boys were born four months premature and each weighed not much more than a pound. They are so tiny; their feet are no bigger than a postage stamp. I have to hold them with my eyes, as they are too fragile to touch and surely too tiny to survive.

Our babies are in a Neonatal Intensive Care Unit. This is a world filled with alien sounds and strange silences. Alarms beep, ventilators swoosh—but the babies make no sound. They can't cry with tubes down their throats.

A full-term baby is born at about 40 weeks gestation. My babies are born at 24 weeks. Many born this early will die within 48 hours. Of those who survive, more than 80% go home with life-altering issues—such as cerebral palsy; blindness; deafness; lung disease; seizures; learning difficulties; and social disabilities like autism.

I'm terrified my boys will die, but even more so that they might live a life constrained with severe disabilities. What is in store for these two who came too early? What will this mean for their future? For ours?

I kept a journal of this time and my scribbled notes fill several volumes. On days when I was too overwhelmed to write, my mother was there to record the events—and there were many days when I could not write.

Having witnessed this journey of extreme premature birth, I am profoundly changed and find all things in my life are relative to this experience. I see more clearly the humanity and fragility of families everywhere. I know now that hope is ever-present in our lives. Hope is the wisdom that comes from the strength of faith. Hope is the compassionate skill of the medical community. Hope is the never-wavering love of a parent for their child. Hope is ever-present, even when you are told you have none.

Jen Sinconis (aka Mama)

Do They Remember?

My son is 21 months old and he is only just now strong enough to pull himself upright holding on to furniture. Standing at a coffee table, he concentrates on stacking alphabet blocks one atop the other—ignoring the evening news that airs on the TV behind him.

The news coverage is about hospital care. The camera cuts to the scene of a Neonatal Intensive Care Unit where a reporter is interviewing a doctor.

The reporter's microphone picks up the background sound of a ventilator alarm. Instantly my son pulls one arm up across his forehead as if to protect him from danger. Then he slowly turns to stare at the TV.

As he peeks out from behind his arm held like a shield across his face, the newscast shifts to another story. It is only then that my boy exhales deeply and resumes his play.

Does he remember?

I hope not.

Journal

"The world of Neonatal Intensive Care
is both frightening and reassuring.
It is a world of anguish and of pure joy.
It is a world that offers hope,
but promises none."

Michele M. Kemper

Chapter 1 - *There's Two in Here!*

"God touched our hearts so deep inside
our special blessing multiplied."

Unknown

Thursday, June 8, 2006

I am delighted with my first pregnancy. My husband Justin and I have this as part of our master plan. College is behind us. Our wedding album has gathered three years of dust, and our careers are underway. We have our retirement account established, ample living expense stashed in a savings account, and a house in the suburbs. Just like the rest of our lives, this pregnancy falls nicely into its assigned place.

Justin leaves work early and joins me for a routine OB-GYN appointment and our first ultrasound. I am so excited to get a picture of our baby.

As I lay on the exam table, the lab tech studies the image on the display. Her prolonged silence makes me extremely nervous.

"Is there something wrong?" I ask.

"Hum…well…hum…everything looks fine," she stammers.

I look past her shoulder to the image displayed on the monitor. It reminds me of something I saw in a pregnancy textbook. As I point at the two fuzzy white smears on the screen I ask, "Is that what I think it is?"

"Yes," she says with a laugh. "You definitely have two of them in there!"

Justin and I sit in shocked silence.

I'm in such a daze, when we leave the exam room I walk right into a seven-foot tall sign knocking the entire display to the floor with a loud crash.

Twins! Oh my gosh! Then I grin.

***

Dr. Umber, my OB-GYN tells me this is a high-risk pregnancy because my twins share a single placenta. I listen to him explain a list of concerns, including twin-to-twin transfusion syndrome[1] and the issues that can arise when two babies share one placenta.

I am sure these problems won't happen to me, as I am healthy. I am not a smoker, gave up my occasional glass of wine and don't do drugs—heck, not even aspirin.

I tell myself, *I will have a normal pregnancy and grow delightfully huge with twins.* That's my plan, or so I naively think.

Dr. Umber excuses himself to take a phone call. While he steps away briefly, I daydream about the exciting changes twins will bring to our household.

***

Our house has been full of pets since...well, forever. We have a dog and two cats and they've been my 'babies' up to this point.

I can't imagine a household without the love of pets; however, I do think ours have been conspiring lately to create as much chaos as they can before the twins come.

Just yesterday the cats climbed into the china hutch and knocked over the wedding glassware, and Jameson the dog chewed a big hole in one of the cushions of our brand new La-Z-Boy sofa.

Jameson is a mix breed of Boston and Staffordshire terrier. This kind of terrier is referred to as a 'nanny dog' in England where the breed originates. We worked hard to socialize Jameson when he was a puppy, and I am confident he'll be a great companion for our twins.

---

[1] Twin-to-twin transfusion syndrome (TTTS) refers to a range of conditions that affect identical twin pregnancies when the babies share a single placenta. The shared placenta contains abnormal blood vessels that connect the umbilical cords and circulation of the twins. Placental sharing refers to how much the single placenta provides each twin with oxygen and nutrients needed to thrive in the womb. Unequal sharing can cause serious development issues and can be a life-threatening condition for one or both babies.

***

Dr. Umber returns to the exam room and continues his update on what to expect when carrying identical twins.

"The babies are inside a single amniotic sac and share a single placenta. This is called a monozygotic twin. It's not hereditary—just a fluke of nature where a single fertilized egg splits into two embryos. And because your babies come from a single egg, they share virtually the same genetic code."

He flips open a big calendar on his desk and adds, "The split of a single egg into two embryos occurs sometime during the first two weeks after fertilization."

With a brief glance at the calendar, I mentally count back the days and realize Justin and I were vacationing on the sunny beaches of Mexico when our babies first became two.

The doctor concludes his 'mom of twins' speech saying, "A single baby is usually carried for a full 40 weeks. Twins however, tend to come earlier—around 36 weeks."

Hey, I can ace this. I expect to carry my babies to their full term due date!

***

The shock of finding out we are having twins has not worn off. I find myself mentally wandering off topic at work as I try to come to grips with what twins will mean in our lives.

Justin takes some time to process this too. He is worried about how we can afford two babies at the same time. This means double daycare expense and funding two in college at the same time.

We always planned to have two kids; just not all at once. Twins mean we will complete our family in one fell swoop.

As the shock starts to wear off, I discover I love being pregnant. I am even more excited when at 20 weeks gestation I learn we're having boys!

Each day I pour over books to learn everything there is to know about pregnancy. I read about the stages of fetal development and relish knowing my sons are growing inside me. Safe. Healthy. Protected. Loved.

My biggest worry right now is how I will tell my identical twins apart.

Tattoo? *No.*

Piercing? *No.*

I know; I'll use a permanent marker and write their names on their big toe!

Chapter 2 - *Emergency Delivery*

"We must accept finite disappointment,
but we must never lose finite hope."

Martin Luther King, Jr.

Monday, October 9, 2006
NICU Day 1

I t's the middle of the night and I can't sleep. I am usually awakened as the babies jockey for new positions in the ever-decreasing space they share in the womb. This is typically a comforting way to wake up, but tonight it is not the movement of the twins I feel—rather it is strange pains across my belly and lower back that wake me. Guess this must be the Braxton-Hicks false labor I read about in the pregnancy textbooks.

The illuminated face on the bedside clock shows 4:45 AM. The pains haven't let up, so I figure it's about time to call the doctor. It is probably nothing, but best to check just in case.

Trying not to wake my snoring husband, I roll awkwardly to get out of bed and waddle downstairs. I put on a pot of decaf coffee and place a call to Dr. Umber's office.

***

Normally I would be commuting downtown to my job as a marketing analyst with a financial services firm, but for the past week I've been working from home. My doctor told me to stay off my feet now that the pregnancy is entering the third trimester.

I plop down on the sofa avoiding the cushion Jameson devoured. Trying to balance a laptop on my mountainous belly, I dial in to my office.

Today I have a full schedule of conference calls with our sales staff. Even though it's 5:00 in the morning here on the west coast, these calls are with our eastern offices— so I am able to get an early start on the workday.

Between these conference calls, I squeeze in one to the doctor's office and leave a voice message asking, "Who the hell is Braxton-Hicks and why does he hurt so much?"

Justin heads off to work, and I wave goodbye with the phone glued to my ear.

As I juggle my work calls, the doctor's office phones back. They want me to get to the hospital right away to be checked out.

I let my co-workers know I am going to run in for a quick check-up with the doctor, but I expect to be back in time for the afternoon conference call.

Since I can't comfortably fit behind the steering wheel and probably shouldn't drive while having these darn pains, I call Dad for a ride. He's retired; so if he isn't already on the golf course he should be available to fill in as chauffeur.

***

As Dad drives me to the hospital, the pain becomes unbearable. I grab my cell phone and speed-dial Justin.

"Honey, you need to meet us at the hospital. I think something is wrong."

As soon as we arrive at the Emergency Room, I am rushed to the Birthing Center where Dr. Umber administers a dose of magnesium sulfate to hold off labor. This horrible stuff makes my blood feel like it is on fire. Right now, this fierce burning sensation in my veins hurts worse than the titanic waves of labor pain. We'll find out much later I am having an allergic reaction to these drugs.

***

The large wall clock shows 1:48 PM and the medical team is winding down their activities in my room. On the way out, one of nurses pats my arm and says, "Sweetie, the drugs are doing their job—your labor has stopped and you can look forward to a nice long bed rest."

Bed rest? My pregnancy still has 16 more weeks to go! How can I possibly stay in bed for nearly four months?

I don't have long to dwell on this. Just minutes after she leaves the room a hot wave of pain washes over me. Blood gushes from between my legs and fills the bed.

Oh my God. It feels like a baby is trying to push his way out.

I grab Justin's hand and yell to Dad, "Go. Get help. Now!"

A nurse rushes in, takes a look at me and smacks her palm against the emergency page button on the wall above my head. In one continuous flow of motion, she pulls up the side-rails of my bed and throws Justin a pair of scrubs.

I glance over at my husband and see in his confusion he has the scrubs on backwards. I can't help but smile. How can my brain register this diversion as humor in the midst of such fear?

The doctors and nurses literally run as they push my bed down the hallway to the Operating Room. The speeding bed breaks a hand sanitizer dispenser off the wall, and my mind records this frenzied race as if everything is happening in slow motion.

Mom has a long drive to get here from her corporate headquarters where she is an executive officer with a financial services company. She arrives at the hospital just in time to see this mad bed race. As my bed careens past, I look up and lock eye contact with my mother. She has a fraction of a second to take in this scene as a wave of panicked recognition spreads across her face.

In the Operating Room, Justin barely finishes telling the anesthesiologist what I am allergic to when a nurse tells him that he has to leave. Things are so hectic to get the surgery moving they don't have time to do a full prep—just get the anesthesia in and start the C-section.

I remember watching the nurse lather me in betadine and the doctor holding the scalpel above my belly.

"Hey, I'm still awake!"

I don't feel pain—just a wave of dread as I hold my breath for what is to come.

The anesthesiologist leans forward and speaks something in my ear, but I am asleep before I can sort out his words.

***

Outside the Operating Room, Mom and Dad stand vigil with Justin. Mom recalls the details for me later.

The loudspeakers are paging the names of doctors to come to the OR—*Stat!* Doctors in surgical garb run the long hallway towards the Operating Room, tying up their facemasks in mid-stride.

More urgent pages pour from the loudspeakers calling for lab supplies and blood. Justin slumps to his knees as a lab tech runs past holding three large packets of blood.

The hospital Chaplain comes to stand with my family. Mom says his presence is more disquieting than comforting. She is sure he has come because the hospital expects to deliver bad news.

***

Dr. Umber's assistant surgeon finally comes out of the OR and says, "Jen is going to be okay. It appears that the placenta tore and separated from the uterus. That's why she hemorrhaged and went into labor so quickly. Jen will be taken to a recovery room shortly and the babies have been placed in the NICU[2]."

He says nothing more about the babies. Instead, he turns to the Chaplain and almost whispers, "I think now is a good time for you to take the family to see the babies."

---

[2] Neonatal Intensive Care Units (NICU) were developed in the 1950-60's by pediatricians to provide specialized care for premature newborn infants. These units are typically directed by one or more neonatologist, and are staffed with nurses, nurse practitioners, physician assistants, resident physicians, respiratory therapists, and other ancillary services necessary for the care of critically ill newborns.

Mom wonders if the doctor is giving our family a chance to say goodbye to the twins. How could they possibly survive being born nearly four months early? Before moving on to a career in business, my mother was a nurse in the mid 1970's. What she remembers from this time as a nurse is that babies born 16 weeks premature don't survive.

The Chaplain shows my family to the NICU—or 'nick-you' as it is pronounced. After presenting ID, they are allowed to enter through a set of security doors.

Just inside the doors are sinks where everyone scrubs in with antiseptic soap. The Nurses' Station is in the center of the NICU, surrounded by two-dozen patient rooms. Each room holds one or two babies, and most of the rooms are the same size—about 12-by-14 feet with a small two-person sofa bench along the back wall. The rooms are packed full of high-tech medical equipment—isolettes, monitors, computerized IV poles, ventilators, x-ray machines, and much more.

Babies needing urgent care right after birth are placed in the largest of these NICU rooms. It's about 30-by-30 feet—but even this large room can feel cramped when it fills up with doctors, sub-specialists, and state of the art medical equipment.

Our hospital refers to this large room as 'The Quad' since it is big enough to hold four isolettes[3]. There's a window smack in the middle of the wall connecting the Quad to the Operating Room. It looks like a McDonald's drive-up window; and it is through this window that a

---

[3] Isolette is an enclosed clear-plastic infant bed that provides a heated and humidified sheltered environment for babies that are too small or too sick to maintain their own body temperature. Access to the baby is via armholes in the sides of the isolette or by lifting the lid. Early versions were called incubators. There are various models of isolettes with differing features, but for simplicity this journal refers to all of them collectively as *isolette*.

critically ill newborn is passed to the waiting arms of the Level III[4] NICU team.

***

My babies are born at 2:39 and 2:40 PM. The first one born is called *Baby A*. He cries immediately after birth, and his coloring is a poor cyanotic blue. He weighs 800 grams (about 1 lb. 14 oz.) and is delivered by emergency C-section in a breech position. This is the little one that was trying to push his way out.

The second one born is called *Baby B*. He weighs in at a scant 674 grams (about 1 lb. 7 oz.). This baby is cyanotic and flaccid. He does not cry. He is not breathing.

The Apgar test is given right after the birth in the delivery room. This test is used to evaluate a newborn's physical condition and to determine if there is immediate need for extra medical or emergency care. The scores can range from zero to 10. A low score means the baby is in need of additional emergency medical attention.

At one minute after birth, *Baby A's* score is 5 and *Baby B's* score is 2.

***

---

[4] Nurseries are rated on three levels. Level I is a healthy newborn nursery—largely nonexistent today because mothers and healthy babies have a short hospital stay and often share the same room. Level II is an intermediate or special care nursery for a baby born prematurely or suffering from an illness. These babies may need supplemental oxygen, intravenous therapy, special feedings, or more time to mature before they can be discharged. Level III admits babies who cannot be treated in either of the other two nursery levels. These babies may be small for their age, premature, or sick full term infants who require advanced medical care such as ventilators, special equipment, or surgery. The Level III units are typically found in a large general hospital or as part of a children's hospital.

My family, along with the hospital's Chaplain, is lined up along the back wall of the Quad room where they watch the doctors feverishly work to resuscitate our babies.

One baby struggles to breathe and one is not breathing at all. The outlook is grim.

Dr. Placket is intubating *Baby A* to help him breathe with the aid of a ventilator[5], while Dr. Lesotho tries to intubate *Baby B*. The tube won't go down *Baby B's* throat—so Dr. Lesotho is manually bagging oxygen for the first three minutes of life as he tries to force air into the lungs.

As soon as Dr. Placket gets *Baby A* intubated and on a ventilator, he turns to *Baby B* and takes over for Dr. Lesotho. Intubating the second boy is nearly impossible. After several tries, he is able to get the ventilator tube in place. Now both babies are on an oxygen machine to help them breathe.

***

Dr. Placket an athletic looking man in his late 50's. He stands about six feet tall with shockingly blue eyes and a stock of thick silver-blonde hair poking out at odd angles from under his surgical cap. His movements are fluid with no wasted energy—like an Aikido grand master. As he works silently to resuscitate the babies, the medical team surrounding him quickly performs a series of tasks. It's as if they are responding to his unspoken commands. We'll find out later Dr. Placket is the Director of the NICU and has been practicing medicine for well over 30 years.

The other neonatologist is Dr. Lesotho. His dark-espresso physique stands over six feet seven inches, with long legs that call to mind a track runner on an Olympic

---

[5] A ventilator mimics natural breathing as it pushes air in and out of the lungs. This type of oxygen therapy involves a tube placed into the baby's airway to administer breaths to keep the lungs expanded. A computer measures how much gentle pressure the ventilator needs to push the oxygen in and to pull carbon dioxide out.

team. The doctor's angular face looks 40-something, and we will learn he has been working in NICU settings for over ten years.

***

Dr. Lesotho stands in the middle of the Quad room eyeing the monitors above each isolette, quietly calling out for updates on meds and vital readings. He turns and sees my family huddled in the corner of the room and steps over to them.

"I am Dr. Lesotho." His Queen's English accent carries a lilt of South Afrikaner as he pronounces his name *leh-soo-too*.

"These babies have severe breathing complications. I am sorry."

He pauses as if to gather his thoughts, and then continues with a melodic accent. "I assure you I have much experience and I have seen many babies born too soon."

Pressing his palms together with fingertips pointing up, Dr. Lesotho speaks into his clasped hands held close to his lips.

"These babies are very fragile. I tell you this so you know what you face. I will try my best to help these babies—but they are most fragile. Please. Know this."

One of the medical team interrupts Dr. Lesotho with an update on *Baby B's* status. The doctor quickly turns back to my family and with an air of urgency he asks, "Who is this baby's father? Your baby is hemorrhaging. I must have permission to give your baby blood."

Justin takes a small step forward and in a near silent voice says, "I am."

After several minutes pass, Dr. Lesotho again approaches the family. He stares down intently into their faces as if to judge whether they will comprehend what he is about to say.

"We know some babies born this early will survive, but if there are severe lung issues the survival rate drops to

20%. Of those that do survive, 80% will have long-term problems."

"What do you mean by problems?" Mom asks.

"There will be problems with motor skills like cerebral palsy, hearing and vision problems, and lung issues. There may be difficulties learning math, forms of autism, or other social development issues."

The statistics are mind numbing. Mom grabs hand towels to use as notepaper to record these conversations. These paper towels will eventually become the first pages of our NICU journal.

***

The Chaplain gently touches Justin's shoulder.

"Would you like me to baptize the babies now?" he asks.

It is clear survival is questioned and Justin is too overwhelmed to form words. So closing his eyes and with a slight nod of his head, he gives approval.

"What else can I do to help your family?" the Chaplain asks.

Mom tells him, "I must have a picture of each boy for my daughter. She must have a picture of her babies..." She stops short of saying, *before it is too late.*

***

Twenty minutes have passed since blood was ordered for *Baby B.* Dr. Lesotho demands of the nurses, "Where is this blood?"

More time passes and still there is no blood delivery. The doctor turns to Nurse Modra—a petite, dark-eyed woman in her late 30's with warm café au lait skin—telling her with a calm measured tone to call the lab.

"Tell them I must have the blood now or this baby will not survive."

The blood is finally delivered. With a quick glance at the packaging label, the doctor sees it is past-dated. The blood product is at the end of its shelf life and must be tossed out.

Dr. Lesotho spits out his words; "You tell them they are killing this baby! If they do not deliver blood immediately, they are responsible for this baby's death!"

Our world has crash-landed. This is too much to bear.

***

I awake in the recovery room and glance at the clock. It says 5:30 PM. Even though there are nurses milling about, I feel so alone. No family. No babies.

The doctor allows Justin to come see me, and he pulls the curtain around my bed as if to give us a measure of privacy.

I ask Justin how the babies are doing.

All he will say is, "Honey, they are so tiny—so very tiny."

I know he is holding back, but I am woozy from the anesthesia and do not probe with any more questions. In fact, I am so out of it I don't feel anything. I have no worries. I have no feelings of any kind. I can't comprehend what has happened.

***

Back in the NICU, Dr. Lesotho steps over to speak with my family once again.

"I am much concerned for *Baby B*. It is possible your baby has a brain hemorrhage. This large machine you see here is to check for bleeding in the brain."

The doctor flashes a forced smile and repeats his earlier prognosis. "If your babies survive, you must know they have an 80% chance of long-term problems."

The words hit like a tidal wave. Hope drains from the room.

Is the doctor trying to prepare us for a decision on whether we continue heroics? Dad takes my father-in-law aside to talk about what might be facing our family tonight. He wants *all* of the family united in their support—as Justin and I may face the hardest decision of our lives; one too dreadful to even put into words.

***

In the NICU, Mom is still on her mission to find a camera. She recruits one of the nurses to help her with the search. The nurse digs out a dilapidated Polaroid from a supply cabinet and takes a picture of each boy. The quality is so poor you can hardly tell the photo is of a baby.

Mom carries the two instant photos to me as if they are the crown jewels. These pictures are the closest I will get to my sons for the next 24 hours.

***

It's nearly 10:00 PM and my family gathers once again around my recovery bed. They look so worried. I try to act positive to raise their spirits. I can't figure out why everyone is so emotional.

The only thing they will say is, "The babies are tiny."

What's the big deal about being tiny?

No one has said a single word about how serious all this is.

Mom shows me the hand towels she has been using as notepaper. She reads aloud a few carefully censored excerpts, and I hear my babies referred to as *Baby A* and *Baby B*.

Justin and I decided on names long ago. *Baby A* will be named Aidan and *Baby B* is Ethan. The names are assigned in this sequence simply because the "A" in Aidan aligns with *Baby A*.

As we name our sons, it dawns on us—we all have new names! Today Justin and I are Daddy and Mama. My mother becomes Nana and Dad is Papa. New names cascade through both sides of our families, turning brothers into uncles, sister-in-laws into aunts, and parents into grandparents.

Before leaving for the night my mom, now known as Nana, goes to each boy and whispers their name to them—promising they will meet their mother in the morning.

***

I study the fuzzy Polaroid pictures of my sons taped to my bed rail—but all I see are blurry images.

Emotion washes over me. I failed them. I failed to carry my babies to term. I feel cheated. I had my pregnancy taken from me and I lost out on the final trimester.

I am angry. The moment I had looked forward to for so long has been stolen from me.

And I feel guilty for focusing so much on what I lost. I should be focused on my babies. What have they lost?

Chapter 3 - *Mama, Meet Your Sons*

"Hope begins in the dark,
the stubborn hope that if you just show up
and try to do the right thing the dawn will come.
You wait and watch and work;
you don't give up hope".

Anne Lamott

Tuesday, October 10, 2006
NICU Day 2

I ask the nurses to keep my door closed. I want to block the sound of laughter and happy conversations coming from the other Birthing Center rooms—but the nurses forget and leave the door ajar each time they enter.

Justin has fallen asleep in the chair next to my bed. He looks exhausted, so I don't wake him to close the door.

***

I have an early morning visitor. It is the hospital's Chief Operations Officer. She has come to tell me she has seen the babies. Apparently my one-pound boys are garnering a lot of attention.

"Your twins are the tiniest surviving babies ever at this hospital!"

I wish this record were not ours.

"You must be so proud of your miraculous boys."

This is weird—she has seen my sons before I have.

"The twins are a high profile case and we're all pulling for you."

What a strange thing to say. I heard the babies are tiny, but isn't this a bit melodramatic?

***

Mom and Dad (I have to remember to call them Nana and Papa now), stop by first thing this morning. After a brief hello, Justin takes them to the NICU to see the twins.

Here I sit, stuck waiting for the doctor to issue orders to let me out of bed. I am anxious to see my babies. If permission doesn't come soon I am going AWOL to find my sons!

Finally, the orders are posted. I am allowed out of bed for 15 minutes every three hours—but only on the condition that I use a wheelchair. I send an urgent text message to Justin to come get me as I don't want to wait a second longer.

"Hurry! Hurry!" I urge Justin as his pushes my wheelchair towards the NICU.

What I see there overwhelms me. I try to keep my emotions in check; however I feel a wave of panic and denial washing over me. I was told the boys are tiny, but until you see a one-pound baby it's impossible to imagine. I never envisioned them being so small and so incomplete. Their skin is nearly transparent—I can see right through to the veins underneath. They are so incredibly tiny—about the same as a Starbuck's venti-size coffee cup.

My babies are covered with wires and tubes, and cotton padding shields their eyes. Their translucent skin is blanketed with fine downy hair and there is no fat on their bodies. Little bony chests are concave, and heave up and down in the same rhythm as the ventilator forcing air in and out of their lungs.

This is not what a baby is supposed to look like! They look like shriveled aliens with misshaped heads and incomplete bodies.

I don't think of them as mine. I don't feel any attachment for them. I thought I'd feel this great tug of motherhood; instead I just feel empty. I can't process this.

There is an alarming number of medical staff swarming around the babies and the atmosphere is intense. A doctor breaks from this mass to tell me he is giving Ethan a second blood transfusion, and that he's placing him on a high-powered ventilator as the lungs have collapsed.

I don't hear anything else said. It's as if I landed in an old silent movie. The overwhelming sights of the room fade to black and white as I block out all sound.

I just want this to be over.

I want to wake up and be pregnant again.

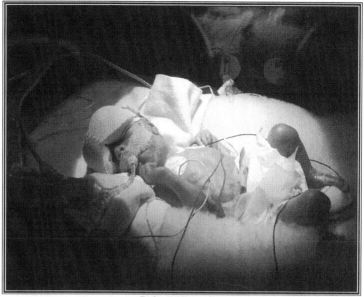

Baby "A" (Aidan)

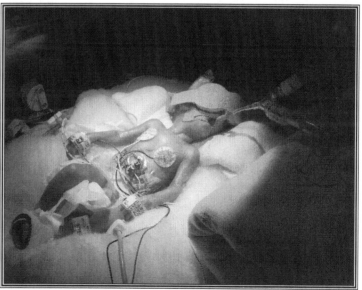

Baby "B" (Ethan)

On my second visit to see the boys, Dr. Lesotho gives an update on what we can expect.

"There are four major hurdles for babies born as premature as your babies. Survival chances will increase when each hurdle is met. The first is to get past the initial 24 hours. Your babies have passed this hurdle."

"The second hurdle is the 48-hour mark. Only 20% of preemies born this tiny with lung issues as severe as your babies survive this long. Of those that do survive, 80% will have some level of permanent disability."

He pauses for a moment; then rushes ahead. "The third hurdle is the 72-hour mark. Many life-threatening issues such as bleeding in the brain and unstable blood pressure problems will arise in the first three days of a preemie's life."

Seeing that we are taking notes the doctor slows his heavily accented speech a bit, and then concludes; "And the last hurdle is the seven-day mark. If no new health issues arise in the first week, survival statistics go up. You understand? Yes?"

We jot down these numbers on the hand towels we're using as notepaper. The odds are overwhelming, and to deal with this we simply tell ourselves, *we will get to the seven-day mark with no new health issues.* This will not be the last time we twist a doctor's cautious words to manufacture our own hope.

***

After a quick break to send email updates to the family, Nana rejoins us in the Quad room.

"Look," she says, "Aidan is on CPAP[6] oxygen support!"

---

[6] CPAP (Continuous Positive Airway Pressure) oxygen therapy is generally used when breathing difficulty is not severe enough to require a ventilator. CPAP uses a nose mask held tightly in place with a strap around the head. It gives air under mild pressure to keep the lungs partially inflated between breaths so as to make breathing easier. While CPAP forces air in, it is up to the baby to exhale on their own.

One of the senior nurses hears us and joins our CPAP discussion. She tells us this support level is less invasive than the ventilator Aidan was on yesterday. The nurse's name is Julie. She's petite and dressed in scrubs with her shoulder-length blonde hair tucked up under a cap. I don't know it yet, but Julie will be one of the nurses I lean on for emotional support throughout this ordeal.

Continuing the discussion Julie says, "CPAP gives air under mild pressure to keep the lungs partially inflated between breaths. And you can see this is done with a mask over the nose rather than a tube down the throat."

She adds one more update. "Aidan has not needed another blood transfusion since last night."

No need for more blood?

This sounds like progress to us, so Nana and I say aloud, "This must mean he is doing better."

Dr. Lesotho overhears us talking to Nurse Julie and interrupts before she can respond. With his heavily accented words he says, "I do not like words 'doing well' or 'getting better' when describing these babies. Babies as fragile as yours are stable or unstable. Babies this premature do not get better for some time. Please. Know this."

His dark eyes search our faces to see if we understand. It will not be until much later that we will truly appreciate the slim margin separating stable from unstable.

***

My 15-minute visit is over. Justin wheels me back to my room in the Birthing Center where we find a constant line of nurses who stop by to chat. They want to meet the mother of the famous one-pound twins. Yesterday everyone avoided me. Now 24 hours have past and people are more at ease talking with me.

I haven't heard the word *'congratulations'* from anyone. While my room is filled with flowers, not a single arrangement looks like it was meant to celebrate the arrival of a baby. These flowers look like bouquets from a funeral parlor. Each one is a thoughtful gift, but I just see them as an expression of '*I am so sorry for your loss.*'

***

This afternoon Nana brings me a new spiral notebook to use as a journal. She copied the updates made yesterday on paper towels into this notebook, and explains how journaling is a useful way to organize information.

I jot down my questions and notes on the boys' condition, along with my thoughts on a daily—if not hourly—basis. While I keep the journal postings current, Nana handles communication with our family and friends by email.

October 10th - email to family:

Jen saw her boys for the first time today. She was able to 'hold' Aidan by reaching through the sides of the isolette and placing one hand gently at the top of his head and the other hand cupping his feet.

Aidan's feet are the size of a postage stamp. His head is about the size of a very small orange. Skin is so fragile it comes off merely by touch. His eyelids won't develop and open for another two or three weeks. He looks like a newborn hairless mouse with eyes fused closed and translucent skin.

Ethan is too fragile to touch. His blood pressure is not stable and he will be given another transfusion of red cells shortly. Both babies bled out while Jen was crashing and Ethan got the worst of it. He is very low on red blood cells to carry oxygen, so the transfusions of packed cells are to stabilize his blood pressure and to carry oxygen to his lungs and vital organs.

Someday, when the boys are in their teens, this will make for very good stories. We will tell them how they gave their daddy and mama a scare by arriving too soon.

However, our focus right now is on the babies growing bigger and stronger…and I think we're going to be at this hospital for quite some time.

Michele (aka Nana)

***

I settle into a wheelchair as Justin pushes me down the hallway towards the NICU for one more visit before bedtime. As we round the corner, the hall is blocked with emergency crash carts. The doorway to our babies' room frames frantic activity of doctors and nurses urgently working on each boy. Alarms are bleeping sharply and above this sound I hear orders for medications being called out and punctuated with '*Stat!*'

As we watch from the doorway, I feel like something is sucking the life out of my babies—an invisible force I can't see and I can't fight. In this instant, a titanic wave of emotion flows into my core. The boys are no longer alien babies lying in isolettes. They are mine. I am to protect them and love them and provide for them.

I reach for Justin's hand. How can we protect our sons? I decide right then, the one thing we will bring to this room every day is *hope*. I will not allow any words of doubt or tears in the room with my boys.

Justin wheels me away so I can cry in private. My babies will not hear my sobs.

Wednesday, October 11, 2006
NICU Day 3

Justin helps me into the wheelchair and once again we navigate the hallways from the Birthing Center to the NICU. At the security door we ring the buzzer for entrance. Lacy, the Health Unit Coordinator lets us in.

She's a young gal of about college age with auburn hair and a constant smile. This welcoming smile is the first thing we see each time we enter the NICU.

Lacy knows us on sight now, so I don't have to show my ID wristband anymore. After a brief hello, we stop to scrub our hands—just like we were shown on the first day.

Another neonatologist rotated on today—the handsome and youthful-looking Dr. Lim. Mom says he reminds her of a younger version of the virtuoso cellist, Yo-Yo Ma—delicate hands, refined, and brilliant. He has the gift of communication that makes you feel like you're the only priority he has when he is talking to you. I'll find out later, despite his youthful appearance, he has been practicing for well over 20 years and is a recognized expert of babies with severely compromised lungs.

I hold back for a few minutes and watch Dr. Lim from across the room. He is leaning into Ethan's isolette and talking softly to my son. I hear him explain to Ethan the procedure that is about to start and I take an immediately liking to this doctor.

Nurses Julie and Modra are back again this morning. They are both as short as my mom—not much more than five feet tall—and the medical equipment dwarfs them. Both nurses look up when I enter the room and we make eye contact. They silently nod their heads as if to say, *all is going as expected.*

I compliment Modra on her beautiful name—it has such a wonderful and unique sound to it. She tells me it means '*healing hand*'. How appropriate.

These nurses quickly become two of my favorites. They are calm and self-assured even in the midst of NICU chaos. Most important to me, they handle my boys with tender caring touch.

***

It seems like I just got here, but my 15-minutes are up and Justin wheels me back to my room. As soon as I return, one of the Birthing Center nurses scolds me for being out of bed.

"Where have you been?" she snaps. "You're being discharged today!"

Doesn't she know I have babies in the NICU?

I start to tell her I can't leave the hospital, but she interrupts before I can finish.

"Well, it is your third day post-delivery—and besides, we need your room for someone that's going to deliver."

What? They're throwing me out?

I can hardly walk because of my C-Section and there's no way in hell I'm going to leave my babies behind in this scary place.

***

Over the past two days we have met three of the many NICU doctors that work here, and find each has a different communication style.

Dr. Lesotho uses a technical approach filled with statistics—neutral and negative, probable and remote. The statistics lean towards the dark-side of averages as he tries to set realistic expectations.

Contrast this with Dr. Lim who uses a holistic teaching approach. He explains the treatment clearly, and with empathy, so we understand how it is geared to resolve each problem. He is frank and yet reassuring at the same time. We learn more from a short discussion with Dr. Lim than we do from hours researching on our own.

And then there is Dr. Placket, the Director of the NICU. He gives just the right amount of technical information and possible outcomes to keep us focused on the task at hand so we're not borrowing troubles from the future. Dr. Placket's vast experience is reassuring and his compassion remarkable. It will be through his deep blue expressive eyes that I will see the first glimmer of hope.

We need all three of these communication styles—but most of all we need hope.

***

At noon I get another 15-minute visit to the NICU. This time I notice right away each isolette has a new nametag. The boys are no longer identified as *Baby A* and *Baby B*.

Hand-lettered brightly colored signs printed with the names *Aidan* and *Ethan* hang on each isolette. These stand out in sharp contrast to the formality of the high-tech equipment and they are the first and only baby-themed decor in the room.

What a nice surprise.

I make a mental note to say *thank you* to Lacy when I see her again, as I'm sure she is the one who made these signs.

***

Back in my room, I support my C-Section suture line with my hands and make my way to the bathroom. The sutures are red and oozing, and I feel flush with a temp.

To my dismay, my belly is covered with a spreading rash and I pass a large blood clot about the size of a baseball. My OB-GYN is called and he diagnoses a uterine infection.

I am not surprised as the C-section was done so quickly there was no time for a full prep.

Antibiotics are started and Dr. Umber says, "You never heard me say this; that IV guarantees you are not going home today."

Good, at least that's one battle we won't have to fight.

***

A social worker stops by with information on Medicaid benefits. She apologizes, saying her handouts are out of date. They are reproduced from old photocopies and are so blurry I can hardly read them.

I don't know what support a social worker provides for NICU families, but this brief meeting is the first and only time I see her.

Her verbal instructions for Medicaid benefits are confusing. I have a hard time relating to this, as I never thought we'd be candidates for government aid. I have a good health insurance policy; so I don't understand why she is so focused on Medicaid.

I listen carefully as she stresses we must file within one week. How to file is the mystery we are left to figure out on our own.

Shortly after she leaves my room the details of this conversation are pushed out of my head. An overriding question crowds every recess of my soul and takes over. *Will my sons survive...and if they do, will they be seriously disabled?*

***

The next visit to the NICU is a parade of Justin pushing me in the wheelchair as I pull along the IV pole on roller wheels. As soon as we enter the boys' room, I overhear a nurse say, "Aidan's blood gas[7] is not good."

---

[7] Blood gas is a test to check for the amount of oxygen, carbon dioxide, and acidity in the blood. The results are used in determining ventilation therapy for the lungs.

I look frantically over at Aidan's monitor display, but I don't understand what the numbers mean. Turning to Dr. Lim, my eyes silently ask him to explain.

"This means carbon dioxide (CO_2) has built up too high in Aidan's blood. CPAP uses gentle pressure to push oxygen into the lungs; but it is up to Aidan to exhale on his own. If not, CO_2 builds up in the blood."

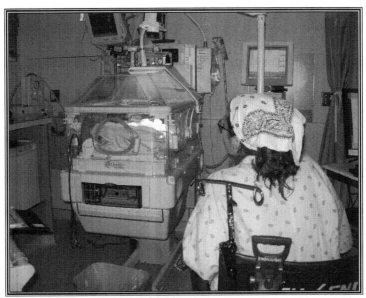

Visiting my sons

"Aidan's lungs are inflated a bit more than I would have liked on CPAP," he continues. "So, I am putting him back on the ventilator for now. This higher level of ventilator support will flush out the excess CO_2."

Dr. Lim switches gears as he moves over to Ethan and places his hand on top of the isolette.

"This little guy was on CPAP earlier—however, his blood gases turned sour right away. Now we have Ethan back on the ventilator as well."

Just as I maneuver my wheelchair next to Ethan, the ventilator red alarm pings frantically.

Dr. Lim glances at my panicked face and says reassuringly, "That's just an alarm to let us know Ethan decided to take himself off the ventilator."

"And we'll just have to see about that," he adds with a smile.

***

Parents of healthy babies learn to recognize sounds of their child's cry. Our preemie babies don't cry—the ventilator tube down their throat keeps them from making any sound at all. So instead, we learn to recognize different alarm sounds.

Everything is monitored—the ventilators; the IVs; oxygen saturation levels; blood pressure; heart rate; body temperature; and so on. Each has its own monitor and own unique alarm sound.

First is the yellow alert with a soft warning *beep-beep-beep*. If the vitals do not return promptly to normal, or if the vitals take a dramatic swing, the alarm escalates to the deep and urgent red alert sound of *BEEP—BEEP—BEEP*.

We will soon be as adept as the medical team in recognizing the source of each alarm.

***

There is no sleeping tonight. The Birthing Center needs my room right now. At midnight they wake me up and hurriedly send me off to a spare room in Pediatrics.

The nurse gives us 'driving directions' to navigate the maze of hallways to find this room. As I sit in the wheelchair, Justin piles my belongings on top of me and we head off to find Pediatrics on our own.

My new room is several floors and two elevator rides from my babies. To get back to the NICU, we will have to go through three sets of locked security doors and wait each time for hospital personnel to buzz us through.

We'll make this long trek every three hours around the clock to deliver pumped breast milk to the NICU freezer and to visit our sons.

Chapter 4 - *Collapsed Lungs*

*"The most important things in the world have been
accomplished by people
who kept on trying when there seemed to be
no hope at all."*

Dale Carnegie

Thursday, October 12, 2006
NICU Day 4

There was no sleep last night—what with moving to a new room at midnight and the racket from the dementia patient in the next bed. My roommate bellowed and hacked up phlegm all night long.

The hospital seems to have packed quite an assortment of overflow patients into the nearly empty Pediatrics wing. I don't know whom I feel more sorry for—me for my isolation from my babies; or the pediatric nurses having to contend with this motley assortment of patients!

Justin once again pushes me in the wheelchair and I hold tight to the portable IV pole dragged alongside. We scrub in when entering the intensive care area; but regardless of how hard we wash our hands, the wheelchair must collect germs as it travels all the way from the Pediatrics wing.

I mean to ask the doctor if the wheelchair could bring germs into the NICU, but I can't keep anything in my head for very long. I add a note to my journal to remind myself to ask about this—however my list of questions grows long and I forget to mention it.

***

The uterine infection is not clearing up and my doctor switches me to another mix of antibiotics. Within the hour, we'll find I am allergic to one of the medications as I break out in massive hives from head-to-toe.

My face looks like a gargoyle and the nurse coats me with an oatmeal-like substance to try to stop the incredibly painful itching.

The hives are now inside my throat and the swelling makes it hard to breathe. I am moved to intensive care where they hook me up to cardiac and respiratory monitors. Now we wait for the hives to subside.

Damn it! This is all I need on top of everything else.

After 16 hours the throat swelling is gone and I insist on being allowed to visit my babies.

Dr. Lim raises his eyebrow when he sees my puffy face still blotchy from the hives. He says nothing as I shrug my shoulders in a silent reply to his unasked question.

***

"Aidan had a quiet day." Dr. Lim says. "The vitals are holding stable and this little guy is tolerating the ventilator."

I'm thrilled when he adds, "Aidan's brain scan came back with no sign of bleeding."

Dr. Lim pauses and sits down on a stool next to me. I sense he has bad news as well.

"Apparently moisture got into the line of Ethan's ventilator last night and caused a partial lung collapse. I put him on the oscillator[8] to try to recruit the collapsed lung tissue."

Oscillator?

Dr. Lim explains the oscillator is the highest level of ventilator support available. The machine keeps the lungs inflated by delivering continuous puffs of air—unlike a regular ventilator that mimics normal patterns of air movement when inhaling and exhaling.

"This is a serious situation. Ethan's blood gas is showing continued problems. I ordered another transfusion to help the red blood cells carry what little oxygen he is getting. If the oscillator doesn't re-open the collapsed lung, we don't have many options."

I understand this means there is no Plan B. I look over at Ethan splayed out in the isolette. His concaved chest does

---

[8] The oscillator is a type of ventilator that delivers a constant series of rapid puffs of oxygen to keep the lungs inflated. It forces air in and out of the baby's lungs at a higher rate than normal breathing and is also known as HFV or High Frequency Ventilation.

not rise and fall—it just vibrates with the rapid puffs of air from the oscillator.

While the update is dark, I do hear a glimmer of good news when Dr. Lim comments on Ethan's latest MRI results. The test shows no bleeding in the brain. I choose to focus on this bit of news as a ray of hope. To me this is a sign that deep inside Ethan there is the will to fight for survival.

***

By mid afternoon I finally get through by phone to the local Medicaid office to file for benefits. Because of the boys' extremely low birth weight, the state considers them to be disabled. I hate the word 'disabled', but if it gets us help with medical bills I'll live with it.

I am not sure what Medicaid entails. I assume this program will pick up balances not paid for by my insurance plan. The NICU bills for two babies are running at $20,000 per day right now…so this is going to be a huge bill. I naively think that between my medical insurance policy and Medicaid all costs will be covered. It won't be until much later that I will earn about the gaps in Medicaid and exclusions in my group health insurance plan that leave substantially large balances in bills for us to pay.

The phone call with the Medicaid office is confusing. I'm told I can't apply until *after* I qualify the babies for Social Security Income (SSI). This is just one more detail missing from the medical social worker's handouts.

After considerable effort, I find the right phone number to call. The SSI phone interview is two hours long!

The SSI rep asks the dumbest questions. "What is Aidan's career? Is Ethan married? What is their income? Do they drive a car…?"

I keep saying, "These boys are five days old!"

The social security rep continues with a list of canned questions before she finally ends up saying; "Your family qualifies for disabled children supplementary income."

"And," she adds with emphasis, "you qualify for the maximum benefit!"

Wow! Maximum benefits!

My bubble of excitement bursts when I learn the benefit for our family is $30 per month, per child—as long as they remain hospitalized. *How will I ever spend it all?*

Before I can ask any more questions, the SSI rep adds a caution.

"You'll need to be sure to keep receipts to prove you spent the money on each boy."

Are you kidding me? I have to turn in a report to prove I spent the $30 monthly checks on the boys when we're racking up $20,000 each day in their hospital bills alone? I don't have time for this nonsense.

***

It must be close to 10:00 PM. The hallway lights are down low and the Pediatrics floor is quiet. I am surprised when my room door opens and a nurse from the NICU comes in to visit.

After a few minutes of idle talk, she stands up as if to leave, then hesitates at the door. Standing there, the nurse awkwardly shifts her weight from leg to leg and seems to have something important on her mind.

Clearing her throat she says, "I think you have incredible strength to handle this situation. I am in awe of your calm in the face of … well, just everything."

She slips in personal advice adding, "Well…ah…I don't think if I had a baby this small I would put them through all this."

I know she means well and is trying to warn me of tough days ahead, and yet this conversation disturbs me. Deep in my soul I wonder if we are supposed to make such a decision.

Y our hives are doing better and the uterine infection is under control," advises Dr. Umber as he pulls the room divider drape closed around my bed. "You can go home today or tomorrow. Your choice."

I want to go home right now. At least at home I can sleep. The dementia patient in the next bed kept me awake again all night long with her constant moaning.

***

I can tell Aidan is having a restless morning. The nurses have to turn him often and suction excess mucus. I wonder if his bruises hurt. Half of his tiny body is covered with deep bruising from internal bleeding. The doctors say this is from being stuck in a breech position in the birth canal for so long. The purple-red discoloration shows up starkly under his translucent skin.

Aidan's ventilator makes an almost inaudible, and yet persistent, clicking sound. A computer controls this ventilator by measuring how much lung energy Aidan generates on his own—then it automatically adjusts the oxygen support pressure accordingly.

I stare at the monitor and watch the display numbers go up and down as the computer makes continuous adjustments in vent support. The numbers show the ventilator is breathing for Aidan about 40% of the time. I turn this into good news—this must mean 60% of the time Aidan is attempting to inhale on his own power.

***

Ethan is still on the oscillator. His CO_2 numbers are way too high. So high, this cannot sustain life and has to be gotten under control. They are giving him another blood transfusion in hopes it will improve his oxygenation level.

Shortly after the transfusion, Ethan's CO_2 blood gas reading drops from the earlier extreme high of 80% down to 46%, and by evening it nudges down to 43%. His lungs are still not exhaling CO_2 properly, but at least the numbers are headed in the right direction.

Ethan is surprisingly active. His arms and legs twitch, jostling his tubes and IVs, which trigger multiple alarms. His hands, supposedly held still with Velcro straps, wiggle and this slight motion manages to dislodge the main lead wires on his tummy, which in turn sets off another series of alarms. We call him the NICU Houdini Escape Artist.

Nurse Modra is so used to Ethan setting off alarms, she simply walks over to his isolette, peers inside, and asks with mock concern; "Ethan, what the heck are you up to now?"

***

I am living in a world of medical terms and I wish I had studied the metric system closer in school. Acronyms are creeping into my everyday language. I now know the jargon for CLD, IVH, and PDA[9]. I can read the monitor screens and find I actually understand some of the numbers. My ears are attuned to the alarms and I recognize the source without looking up to see which of the many monitors are beeping.

There is so much to take in. When the information is confusing, I just turn to Nana and ask her what the term means.

She jokes and says, "I forgot most everything I learned in nurses' training—and heck, it was so long ago I swear we used leeches for routine treatment!" However, it doesn't take long for my mom to slip back into the medical jargon of a hospital setting.

---

[9] Chronic lung disease (CLD), intraventricular hemorrhage (IVH), and patent ductus arteriosus (PDA). I'll describe these conditions in more detail in upcoming chapters.

***

The privacy rules make it hard to meet other parents, however I did manage to introduce myself to a couple of families here.

Lisa and Charlie's twins were born two days before Aidan and Ethan. Their babies weighed just over four pounds each, and fortunately are doing well. Lisa says the doctors expect they'll be out of the NICU in a few weeks.

Until now, it never occurred to me that some babies come and go through the NICU experience with different medical issues and length of stay. I just assumed everyone had the same roller-coaster experience as our family.

While the health issues and the length of stay vary, our hopes and fears are the same. Lisa and I share our experiences and our struggles to parent a NICU baby. Our friendship started at a stressful time in our lives, and we have remained dear friends ever since.

Having another parent to talk to is important. The doctors and nurses are great—but there are some issues only another NICU parent can understand.

Saturday, October 14, 2006
NICU Day 6

The phone rings constantly and my email is overflowing. Family and friends reach out to me— but I can't talk and I can't respond to email. Just saying the words aloud makes this all too real.

Luckily, Nana solves my communication problem. During one of her nighttime wanderings on the Internet, she came across *CarePages.com*. This site provides an easy to use template for creating a web page, and hosts the websites for families in the midst of a medical crisis.

Nana becomes the communication hub for our family. She sets up our website and sends out the first of what becomes a yearlong series of medical updates and photos. From the very first posting, the in-box is overflowing with messages of love, faith, and caring. The words sustain me, and when times are especially dark I re-read the messages from friends and family knowing I am not alone.

The circle of support is immeasurable. As our story spreads, I get messages of hope and prayer from families I have never met—some as far away as England, Australia, Israel, and even one from Croatia.

Motherhood is the international language of mankind. When one mom hurts for her child, we all hurt.

***

The boys are six days old today. Just one more day and we'll be at the seven-day mark. While we know it's not rational, we think if the babies make it to this milestone, it will be like crossing a magic line and nothing but good news will flow. This has been so hard I can't imagine it could get any worse.

***

The boys are receiving their third in a series of drug treatments to close the patent ductus arteriosus (PDA). The cardiologist did a heart scan and found a wide-open PDA. It's of concern; however there is optimism the medication will close this blood vessel.

The doctor explains the ductus arteriosus in an unborn baby allows blood to bypass the lungs since it receives oxygen from the mother and not from breathing air. In full-term babies this blood vessel closes shortly after birth as the baby's blood starts to circulate from the heart to the lungs. However, this vessel frequently stays open in premature babies. When this happens, excess blood flows into the lungs and can cause a series of problems.

The PDA is often treated with drug therapy—and this is successful about 80% of the time. However, if this fails, the ductus may still spontaneously close without intervention. If not, surgery may be required.

***

My hope to make it to the seven-day milestone comes unraveled. The moment I enter the NICU, a nurse jumps up saying; "Tomorrow morning they will likely transfer your boys to Mercy Hospital for PDA surgery."

Heart surgery?

Their hearts are the size of a nickel!

How can this be?

This nurse is on loan from another hospital. I have not met her before, however I quickly figure out she is a 'by-the-numbers' gal. She even insists on referring to the boys with their birth-order names of *Baby A* and *Baby B*.

I privately call her 'Nurse Alarm', because every time she opens her mouth she alarms me. She gives no warning when she blurts out her latest pronouncement of dire outcomes. It's like walking into an ambush. I feel physically beat up just talking to her.

Today my babies are one week old and I have yet to hug or kiss either one. They are a world away from my arms as they lay inside their plastic isolettes. They are so fragile I can't hold them. Just touching an extremely premature baby can be disruptive and overload their systems. So all I can do is hold them in my heart.

***

Dr. Lim is in charge of rounds this morning and starts in our room first.

"I am concerned with Ethan's lungs," he says. "I have him on the oscillator, the highest form of respiratory support available, and this is still not able to keep his lungs from collapsing further. I put Ethan on a morphine drip to take the edge off and to keep him calm so he doesn't overtax his lungs."

I want to joke and ask if he has something to take the edge off for me—something preferably alcoholic and on ice—but this situation is so dreadful I can't say anything lighthearted.

The doctor continues with his update.

"Ethan's platelet count is low, so we'll give him another blood transfusion today."

I look at my journal postings and as my eyes scan the pages I count on my fingers—this is the fifth blood transfusion. Seems a bit odd to count these, but it gives me something to focus on. I am starting to feel like a neurotic-compulsive obsessed with counting things. This ritual of tracking transfusions gives me a sense of order.

***

Nurse Alarm is back again this afternoon. We got off to a bad start yesterday and I hope today will be better.

I greet her with, "Good afternoon."

In response, her words rush out and tumble over themselves.

"*Baby A's* blood pressure is unstable. This is being treated with dopamine and dobutamine. The dopamine dose is at 15 MICs—the highest setting that can be given to a preemie. These steroids are to improve the blood-pumping ability of the heart. When the blood pressure falls below a certain level, the concern is some parts of the body—such as the brain—won't get enough blood and oxygen. His blood gas reading is okay right now, but that is only because the oscillator is on a very high setting."

These words pour out of her so fast I have to struggle to keep my mental balance. Before I can ask a question, she continues her machine-gun burst of dire warnings.

"If this oxygen therapy does not work there is nowhere else to go. The oscillator is cranked up to a very high setting. If he is still not getting a good exchange of CO_2 and O_2 it might be because of the wide-open PDA. This could also be causing his blood pressure to drop precipitously. I think he'll be sent for PDA surgery soon."

Here she goes again. At break-neck speed we have gone from *"Good afternoon"* to *"Your son is in dire need of heart surgery."*

I want to smack her.

Taking refuge from Nurse Alarm, I join Nurse Modra as she tends to routine tasks. She lets me participate and I learn a new skill when she demonstrates how to take my boys' temperature.

Sensing I need more hands-on time with my sons, Modra next shows me how to change their diapers. I find it a bit surprising that there is actually a Pampers™ disposable diaper made for babies this small. It's the size of a folded cocktail napkin—however even this tiny diaper is still too big for my boys.

Each wet diaper is weighed on a scale so the nurses can determine how much fluid goes in and how much comes out.

The boys are so fragile this routine task terrifies me. However, once I learn this, I feel a little bit smug that I can do at least one normal mommy thing—changing a diaper.

Now at last, I feel like their mama and not a visitor.

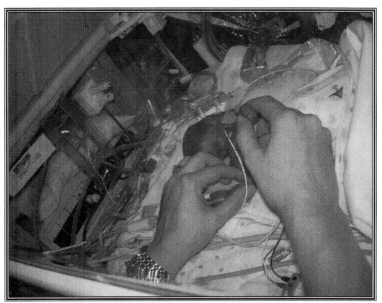

Mama taking Ethan's temperature

As the evening wears on, Aidan continues to be unstable.

Nurse Alarm pipes up again. "The doctors can't give this baby a fourth round of meds to close the PDA—so he will have to be sent to Mercy Hospital for surgery."

My God! Does she get a commission for every PDA surgery?

Despite Nurse Alarm's predictions, the doctor orders a fourth round of medication as he follows a 'wait and see' strategy.

***

I grab a ready-made sandwich in the cafeteria and when I return, I see Nurse Alarm is changing the monitor read-out screen over Aidan's isolette to a new format. When she steps away and a different nurse comes to check, the monitor is switched back to the hospital standard setting.

Nurse Alarm returns, and once again she re-sets the monitor to a different format.

The monitor is flipped back and forth so many times I am on edge.

I pull Nurse Alarm aside and quietly ask, "Can you leave the monitor format on the standard setting? This way I can read them and know how my babies are doing."

She dismisses my request saying, "I like them set this way—and besides, you're not supposed to be reading the monitors anyway."

I've had it!

Nana finds an opportunity to talk privately with Dr. Lim.

"This nurse's communication style might not be a good match for what our family needs right now," she explains.

Dr. Lim nods and says he understands. Nothing more is said, but we never see Nurse Alarm assigned to our babies again.

The day ends on a depressed note with my emotions barely in check. I am having anxiety attacks whenever I leave the hospital. With so many threats of death, I feel as if a part of me has already died.

Chapter 5 - *Brain Bleed*

"Things never go so well that one should have no fear,
and never so ill that one should have no hope."

Turkish proverb

Monday, October 16, 2006
NICU Day 8

When I arrive this morning, I notice two emergency crash carts have been moved into the boys' room—one by each isolette. Dr. Lim notices my wide-eyed panic as I take in the scene. He tells me to just ignore the carts.

"It was a rough night, but I am sure the carts won't be needed today. Last night both babies had lung failures and continue to be unstable this morning."

"But we are making progress," he adds quickly. "They are fighters and the stats are starting to turn the right direction. We were even able to get Aidan off the oscillator and back on the vent."

While Dr. Lim makes adjustments to Ethan's oscillator line, he poses questions to me. "So tell me again; just how far along were these boys?"

"During the last routine exam when I was pregnant, the babies were thought to be just about 24 weeks."

He wonders aloud about this. "These babies present a case for closer to 23 weeks. Their translucent skin; eyes still fused shut; ear cartilage not fully formed—these are all signs typical of 23 weeks. And of course, the seriously underdeveloped lungs are more indicative of 23 weeks."

I studied articles on survival rates at different gestation ages, so this observation is disconcerting. Survival rates drop precipitously for preemies born at 23 weeks.

***

Just before lunchtime, Dr. Lesotho marches in to deliver an update on Aidan's heart. With his unique accent he announces, "The PDA is getting smaller, however it is not closed fully. Please. You must know this. This can re-open."

Dr. Lesotho's tone changes, and he speaks each word so slowly they stand-alone.

"I. Have. Major. Concerns."

I hold perfectly still with every nerve ending tuned to what he is about to say.

"Aidan's blood pressure dropped very much last night and today is unstable. Target pressure is 32 to 38. Aidan's pressure is 38 now, but it was lower last night and he has much need for ventilation. This is not good."

He pauses momentarily, and then repeats himself. "I have much concern for this baby."

These words tighten like a vise on my heart. I know Dr. Lesotho's predictions tend to highlight negatives with more emphasis than positive outcomes. When I ask him how the other doctors view these blood pressure stats, his body language changes. The air between us becomes fragile. I feel I have to filter my questions, or the words will break the very air I am breathing.

After what feels like a full minute of silence, he answers. "Some doctors do not feel this pressure warrants action at this time. But I tell you; this is very much an issue and needs treatment soon. You understand? Yes?"

I can't deal with this right now. I excuse myself with a simple nod of my head. I can't sort through differing opinions when the medical plan is delivered piecemeal. My nerves are in such a raw state I can't think clearly.

***

Ethan had a rough time last night as well, and this morning he continues to desat[10]. This means his ability to regulate his blood oxygen level is unstable. To counter this,

---

[10] Desaturation (desat) refers to a precipitous drop in the blood oxygen level, generally detected by a pulse oximeter. It is sometimes associated with apnea (periods of cessation of breathing) or bradycardia (periods of abnormally slow heart rate).

the doctor cranks up Ethan's oxygen support to 60%—well above standard room air of 21%.

This little guy's respirations continue to be unstable and x-rays show compromised lungs. In fact, x-rays show the lungs are in a state far worse than the doctors expected.

***

I am once again at my usual place perched on a stool with my hands awkwardly thrust through the armholes of an isolette. Every few minutes, I switch back and forth between Aidan and Ethan's plastic boxes.

This is the nearest I can get to my babies. I gently cradle their head with one hand and their feet with the other. The awkward position means my back will ache and my fingers will start to tingle and fall asleep within minutes. With the touch of my fingers, I try to will my boys to fight for their lives.

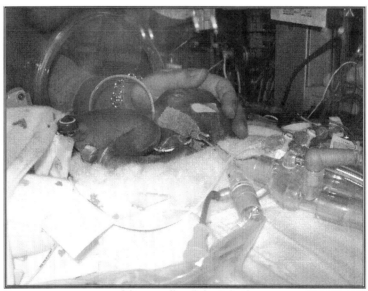

Mama cradling Ethan's head

Normally the light touch of my hands on Ethan soothes him and helps to keep his respirations even—but not today. His breathing is off and he is tripping alarms.

Nurse Modra reacts calmly, even though my heart stops with each red alarm. She checks to see if water has accumulated in the ventilator line, repositions the baby and resets the alarm. She does all this in one continuous motion—so gently Ethan sleeps right through it all.

As Modra adjusts Ethan's monitors, I move over to Aidan's isolette and see him sleeping with one frail leg kicked up across his torso and his tiny arms are outstretched wide. This position looks like his Daddy sleeping—just add the sound of snoring and the picture would be complete.

***

By midday the brain scans are back. Dr. Lim is carefully choosing his words as he explains the results.

"Aidan's scan is clear; however Ethan's shows bleeding in the brain. This bleeding is called intraventricular hemorrhage[11], and the severity is graded on a scale of I to IV."

I hold my breath as he continues.

"Ethan has a Grade II bleed. This did not cause any swelling of the brain, which is good. The bleeding is in the fluid space of the ventricle on the right side, and it is not in the brain tissue itself—which is also very good."

Dr. Lim takes out his pen and draws a picture of a brain and the ventricles on a paper towel—then he marks

---

[11] Intraventricular hemorrhage (IVH) refers to a bleeding in the brain. Blood vessels in the brain of premature babies are immature and fragile. The vessels can be prone to breakage in the first few days after birth when blood pressure and blood flow to the brain tends to fluctuate. The upper part of the brain consists of two hemispheres. Within each hemisphere is a semicircular chamber called a ventricle. The ventricle produces the cerebrospinal fluid, which coats the brain and the spinal column. The ventricles are areas prone to bleeding.

the picture to show me where the bleeding occurred and how this news applies to Ethan.

"Grades I and II are generally considered mild with no long-term effects. Grade III and IV usually have a more serious consequence. Of course this is not something I wanted to see, however it is not unexpected. In a week or so, I will order another brain scan because some bleeds enlarge—but odds are in our favor this will resolve on its own."

I am thankful it is Dr. Lim explaining this to me. I can comprehend bad news more clearly when he delivers it. I hear the devastating words, but they are chosen carefully so as to leave room for hope.

Later, Dr. Lesotho takes Justin and me aside to tell us he has a different opinion on this brain bleed.

"This probably means long-term physical or mental concerns such as cerebral palsy or learning difficulty." He backs this up with an array of statistics to help us comprehend the depth of what we may be facing.

This is too much to handle. I am struggling with fear and can't digest statistics in a meaningful way. His words make me feel like a helpless bystander watching a horrific accident unfold.

Dr. Lesotho delivers more news. "Blood sugar is under control today, but heavy doses of hydrocortisone to control blood pressure can throw this off balance. Pressure is not stable. Your babies continue to have fluctuations. This is not good. You understand? Yes?"

He pauses and searches for the right words. "You must know; many bad side effects come with heavy doses of hydrocortisone...such as deafness. It is worth this risk because we must get blood pressure under control."

"What is causing the unstable blood pressure?" I ask.

"I think this is because of the open PDA. You should know Dr. Lim does not agree. He feels this is because of infection and ordered blood cultures. Now we must wait for lab results."

I leave with a heavy heart.

Chapter 6 - *Crisis Times Two*

"Man can live for about forty days without food,
about three days without water,
about eight minutes without air,
but only for one second without hope."

Unknown

Tuesday, October 17, 2006
NICU Day 9

C risis! It is just after midnight and both boys take a sudden swing into lung failure. Dr. Lim calls Justin and me at home and suggests we come back to the hospital right away. This phone call is beyond terrifying. I don't remember getting dressed or riding back to the hospital. Justin makes this 45-minute drive in less than 25 minutes.

We literally run the hospital hallways to the boys' room where we find Dr. Lim. His solemn expression puts as much fear in me as do his words.

"Ethan's lungs are failing. They may be filling with an infection. Aidan also has a spot on his lungs, and I am concerned he too has an infection."

To make sure we understand the severity he adds, "You may want to call your family now. And if you have a religious leader you would like present, now would be the time. We don't know what will happen over the next few hours."

Justin and I nod in shock and head upstairs where our cell phones have a clearer signal reception to call our families. As we walk out of the NICU, my legs give-way and I crumble into his arms. My pain is unbearable. I can't believe this is happening.

We give each other a pep talk before calling our parents. It's going to be a bad call and we want to sound positive so our families can drive here safely.

That plan goes out the window as soon as I hear my mom's sleepy voice. I completely break down and sob the words; "Mom. Come. They don't think the boys will make it."

***

Both sets of our parents arrive just as Dr. Lim delivers more bad news.

"Aidan's x-ray show his lungs are now in worse shape than Ethan's. I am concerned for both boys."

This is devastating. Emotionally we were not prepared for Aidan's lungs to fail. We had warnings on Ethan for days, but I never expected Aidan to crash. The prognosis is extremely poor. For the first time I acknowledge silently in my heart we may lose them both.

I am unraveling.

We are ushered off to the Quiet Room to grieve. This is a 4x6 closet-size room with a three-person bench and a single chair. On a small shelf is a box of tissue and a discarded brochure titled, "When You Lose Your Baby: A Parent's Grief."

We cram all six of us into this tiny room and everyone is silent with fear. Every part of my body aches and I lean my head on Justin's shoulder and cry. I feel I will never be myself again. The pain is too much.

After a few minutes, I regain my composure and we head back into the NICU room. The nurse tells me Ethan has been given narcotics to keep him perfectly still while Dr. Lim tries desperately to get the ventilator to re-inflate the lungs.

The x-ray display screen shows Ethan's lungs are a solid white mass filled with fluid. Dr. Lim watches this screen as he tries to monitor the progress of the vent tube as it is moved into the lungs. However, the whiteout image of the lungs makes it impossible to see the tubing!

The tension builds as Dr. Lim abruptly pushes the x-ray monitor aside and grabs a hand pump to 'feel his way' into Ethan's lungs. He does this flying blind maneuver by sensing faint lung pressure differences with the hand pump so he knows when the tube is in the optimum location.

If I weren't in such absolute torment, I'd be in awe to watch Dr. Lim's unbelievable skill placing the tube into lungs so filled with fluid.

***

After the longest six hours of my life, Aidan and Ethan's lungs start to re-inflate! This was far too close. Even the normally unruffled Dr. Lim looks wiped out.

Our anguish must be painted on our faces, as Nurse Modra senses our struggle and offers words of comfort.

"I have a decade of experience," she says. "And I have seen many 24-week gestation preemies. What you went through in the past few hours is typical. The NICU is a roller coaster ride of good days and bad days—but it can be survived."

She says all this with a calm and reassuring tone. While no promises are made, I take from her words that other NICU babies have survived similar trauma. I say a silent prayer of thanks for Modra. This is the worse night of my life and her words keep me from tipping into bottomless despair.

My mom is desperate to give me something positive to hang on to. She paints for me a verbal picture saying, "This experience is like riding on the back of a dragon. It's a dangerous ride, and we are scared we'll fall if we let go. So the only choice we have is to hang on tight and tame these dragons not to bite. Your son's are fighting hard to tame the NICU dragons."

This is the first time we call our babies the 'Dragon Tamers.' It seems fitting. This is the fight of their lives.

***

Both boys need extra oxygen support to recruit[12] collapsed lung tissue—but the support won't work if there

---

[12] Recruitment describes the strategy aimed at re-expanding collapsed lung tissue. Mechanical ventilation diverts airflow to the upper regions of the lungs, in contrast to normal breathing where the base of the lungs is better aerated. This means the lower lobes in ventilated patients can collapse and need to be recruited to re-open.

aren't enough red blood cells to carry oxygen to vital organs. Another round of blood transfusions with packed red cells is underway.

By noon the oxygen readings are back within normal range and Dr. Lesotho stops by with his latest pronouncements.

"Blood sugar readings are high—214 in both boys. Normal reading is 150. Since a high sugar reading can be indicative of infection, we need the results from cultures taken yesterday."

He pauses to give his next words the spotlight.

"The lungs are much damaged. But right now I am looking for signs of fungal infection. A fungal infection would be more serious than bacterial—as these are usually fatal in preemies."

How am I supposed to handle this news?

He takes me from lung failure to warnings about fatal fungal infection all in one breath.

I can't think of anything rational to say, so I give voice to the one thought that circles in my heart over and over and ask, "Are they getting any better yet?"

Dr. Lesotho stares at me like I have lost my mind.

I am numb. I've had more pain in one day than my entire lifetime. The last nine days have been rough, but today is the worst.

How will we ever to make it through this? I'm at the edge of collapsing.

I know one thing; I'm not leaving my sons any more. I'll find a place in the hospital to sleep, even if it's on the floor.

***

It has been nearly 24 hours since our families came to stand vigil. Exhausted sets of grandparents are propped on an assortment of chairs and stools throughout the boys' NICU room. There aren't enough chairs to go around, so

Justin leans against the doorframe as if on guard for his sons.

When Dr. Placket walks into the room, we all snap to attention. He has a wide grin spread across his face.

"The lab results are back and they are negative for fungal infection!"

We take a moment to breathe in this good news.

Nana does a double take as she watches Dr. Placket leave the room.

"I know that smile!" she exclaims. "I am pretty sure I met Dr. Placket before…I just can't place him. I have a feeling I knew him long ago."

My mother racks her brain trying to remember where she met Dr. Placket, but she is too tired to pull out old memories.

Wednesday, October 18, 2006
NICU Day 10

Dr. Lesotho catches me in the hallway as I return from the lactation room. He lectures me that I am to give serious consideration to moving the boys for PDA surgery. He says if these were his babies, he would send them to Mercy Hospital.

Transfer? Surgery? What's this all about?

The doctor does not linger to discuss this, so I go looking for reassurance to confirm that the whole team agrees surgery is necessary.

I quickly locate Dr. Lim at the Nurses Station and ask; "What is the team's consensus on PDA surgery?"

Responding firmly he says, "Surgery is out of the question. Your babies are not stable enough to be transferred and would not survive surgery."

His eyes soften and he adds, "Aidan is considered critically ill. His lungs are extremely fragile and we're working hard to keep them inflated."

Dr. Lim knows I am struggling and he takes his time even though I ask the same questions over and over.

I ask again if he thinks a transfer to Mercy Hospital is appropriate.

"No, the boys can not be transferred. Mercy is for surgery while this hospital is for medical management. What the boys need is medical care, not surgery. Besides, they are both on the oscillator and babies cannot be transported on this level of oxygen support."

"To be moved to another hospital their lungs must first be strong enough to survive on a ventilator—that's the highest level of oxygen support that can be used in a transport ambulance."

"The boys are too fragile and unstable right now to even consider moving them. A move is stressful and any more stress on these babies—well, let's just say this would not be a good thing."

Asking the same question from another angle, I probe further. "Once stable would you transfer the boys to Mercy Hospital to help preempt future problems?"

His answer comes quickly, yet is thoughtful. "I am pleased with the amount of stability regained today, and I am confident Mission Valley can handle everything. I cannot justify a transfer because the boys don't have a problem beyond our expertise. And most important, they don't need surgery right now."

I take a deep breath and point out Dr. Lesotho is telling me privately to move the babies to Mercy for PDA surgery right away.

Dr. Lim's eyes widen in surprise, and then close briefly as he gathers his thoughts before responding.

"Dr. Lesotho is relatively new to this area and he is not familiar with how our regional hospitals operate. These babies cannot be transferred to Mercy unless they are going for surgery. And they are most assuredly not candidates for surgery."

***

Returning to the boys' NICU room, I find Dr. Lesotho adjusting an IV line. From his perspective the surgery discussion is apparently not over. He disagrees and will not let this rest. Now he tells me I need to *force* Mission Valley to transfer the boys.

Dr. Lesotho has strong opinions, but I wish he would stop this sideline campaign. I can't keep going back and forth between the attending physicians to sort this out.

I have the utmost confidence in the collective skill of the doctors at Mission Valley. If Dr. Placket and Dr. Lim say it's time to go, we'll go; but for now we stay.

If this weren't so scary, I'd describe this as a TV soap opera. Everyone plays their parts well, but I wish they'd get on the same damn script.

***

The day is not over and Dr. Lesotho has not given up his campaign to transfer the babies. Since Dr. Placket, the Director of the NICU will not order a surgical transfer and I won't force a voluntary transfer, Dr. Lesotho changes tactics. He lobbies my *in-laws* to demand we move the boys.

My in-laws agree with Dr. Lesotho. Now I have my in-laws pressuring me to go against the consensus of the medical team. This division in the family is so disruptive.

When I try to talk to Dr. Lesotho to learn why he feels so strongly about this, I don't know what words to use. I fear I come across as challenging his medical opinion. The air becomes tense. This isn't right. I spend too much time worrying how to phrase my questions.

I know the boys are critical and I know the odds for their survival is low. But I can't help wondering…is this pressure to move the boys to another hospital a defensive move to bring more doctors into the picture? This way if anything does go dreadfully wrong—well, as the saying goes—the boat is packed to spread the responsibility.

I make up my mind to confront Dr. Lesotho and ask him to come only to Justin and me with his medical counsel. Pressuring my in-laws to change our minds is not helpful. It's time to put this to rest. But right now I'm exhausted. I'll do it tomorrow.

***

What a day. I don't dare call my sons' condition stable—but at least they are not crashing. Our families have finally gone home, and Justin left to take care of our pets.

As I sit quietly by the boys' isolettes, Dr. Lim stops by to say hello. No medical updates—just a friendly hello.

"Tonight is a good time for taking pictures," he says.

Seems almost funny to have to be told to take pictures of my babies—and it doesn't take much prompting to unleash the camera.

In the course of taking pictures something special happens. I begin to see the babies as 'my boys' and not as patients. The camera catches what my eyes can't see in the dim light of the NICU. Both boys have red hair! I joke that my sons have more hair than their daddy.

I focus the camera on their little hands and feet—tiny as paper clips. And just for now, what I would have cuddled and kissed and held in my arms, is held by a photo instead.

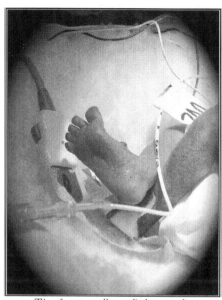

Tiny feet—small as a little paperclip

Thursday, October 19, 2006
NICU Day 11

Dr. Lesotho's accent has curious blend of Queen's English and the poetry rhythm of South Afrikaner. I tell him I find comfort in his voice.

"My maternal grandfather has an accent," I say using my best imitation of Grandpa's Scottish brogue. "He left Scotland after graduating from Strathclyde University where he got his degree as a mechanical engineer. His first job was designing water treatment plants for communities in Nigeria and in South Africa."

With a bit of a laugh I add, "He picked up some of the local languages and he speaks them with a Scottish accent!"

Dr. Lesotho smiles broadly. "I should like to meet your grandfather. Someday? Yes?"

"My family home is in South Africa and my university studies were in England," he continues. "This is where I received advanced training in pediatrics."

I figure now is a good time to talk to Dr. Lesotho about his lobbying efforts with my in-laws. However, this window of opportunity and my resolve both evaporate when red alarms blare and the doctor rushes off to attend to another baby.

***

The boys have been supported with peripheral[13] and arterial[14] IVs for the past 11 days. The IVs have to be

---

[13] Peripheral line is the most common intravenous (IV) therapy. It consists of a short catheter inserted through the skin into a peripheral vein of the arm, hand, foot, leg or scalp. Frequent insertion of IVs can scar the veins making future access extremely difficult or impossible. This situation is known as a 'blown vein', and the person attempting to insert a new IV has to find an access site proximal to the blown area.

swapped frequently as the blood vessels wear down and blow, causing the line to go bad.

The doctors decide it is time now to insert a longer-lasting IV called a PICC[15]. This IV can be left in place longer than other IV types. It is a tricky placement and Dr. Lim wants this done by Nurse Antonia.

"Antonia is the best IV specialist in the area," he says. "If anyone can get the PICC line in these boys, she can."

The plan is to do Aidan's line first. If Aidan does not tolerate this, Antonia will skip any efforts to insert a PICC in Ethan.

Everything goes as planned. Antonia gets Aidan's line inserted with no problems and turns to do Ethan's. His PICC line goes in smoothly as well.

Way to go Antonia!

***

One of the nurses comes to get the boys' weight measurements. This is not an easy task, as neither boy responds well to handling. Another complication is the many IVs, monitor wires, and vent lines—all which need to be suspended to get an accurate weight.

The nurse finishes up and logs Ethan as 660 grams (about 1 lb. 7 oz.). This is down a bit from the 674 grams at birth. Just imagine—Ethan weighs the same as five sticks of butter!

---

[14] Arterial line, sometimes called ART line, uses a thin catheter inserted into an artery and is generally used to monitor blood pressure real-time and to obtain samples for blood gas measurements. An ART line is usually inserted in the wrist, armpit, groin, or foot. With newborns, this line may also be placed through the umbilical cord.

[15] Peripherally Inserted Central Catheter, generally referred to as PICC, is a central venous line placed into a surface vein with the tip of the catheter extending farther into the body until it reaches a large central vein. This line doesn't have to be replaced as often as a peripheral line, so it can be used for long-term treatments.

Aidan's weight is up to 870 grams (about 1 lb. 15 oz.) compared to his 800 grams at birth.

As the nurse finishes posting these weights in the charts she says, "You know…your boys are the tiniest micro-preemies I've ever weighed."

Micro-preemie?

"A micro-preemie is the youngest and smallest of the preterm babies. We use this term to refer to little ones born before 29 weeks."

Our sons, born at 24 weeks and with an extremely low birth weight[16] are among the smallest of the small.

***

The doctors were finally able to turn off the bilirubin (bili) light for both boys today. Yesterday they had a reading of 9.0—but today Aidan's jaundice reading is down to 2.6 and Ethan's is 3.0.

The bili light helps the liver to break down decomposing red blood cells. When the babies are under these bright lights, they wear sunglasses to protect their eyes. The sunglasses are actually tiny cotton pads. Now that the pads are off, we can see Aidan's eyes for the first time. It will be a bit longer before we see Ethan's—they are still fused shut.

Both boys continue to look like newborn hairless mice with translucent skin. No fat and very little muscle; just bones and loose skin.

Precious, *yes.* Pretty, *no.*

***

---

[16] A micro-preemie is the smallest of the preemies, and refers to babies born before 29 weeks of gestation, whereas a pre-term baby is born before 37 weeks and a full-term baby is born at about 40 weeks.

Birth weight is ranked as:

Low Birth Weight: 1500 grams (3 lbs. 5 oz.) to 2500 g (5 lbs. 8 oz.)
Very Low Birth Weight: 1000 g. (2 lbs. 3 oz.) to 1500 g (3 lbs. 5 oz.)
Extremely Low Birth Weight: less than 1000 g. (2 lbs. 3 oz.)

The morning x-ray shows Aidan's lungs are no worse. No improvement, but at least we're not losing ground. His concave chest vibrates from the oscillator's constant stream of rapid puffs of air. I find myself unconsciously breathing with an exaggerated in-and-out rhythm—as if to show Aidan how to mimic a normal breathing pattern.

Ethan's lungs are too fragile to even discuss coming off the oscillator. He occasionally tries to breathe on his own; but still needs more recovery time between each attempt.

***

I ask Nurse Modra to explain the various oxygen treatments. She tells me each level of support has significant differences.

"The highest oxygen support is the oscillator. This machine fills the baby's lungs with puffs of vibrating air. With this therapy the lungs do not contract to expel the CO_2. Instead they are kept constantly expanded with puffs of air."

"The next step down in support is the ventilator. Just like the oscillator, this machine delivers air through a tube placed in the lungs. The big difference is the ventilator mimics normal breathing patterns by expanding and contracting the lungs as it forces the air in and pulls out the carbon dioxide."

"CPAP is the third step down in oxygen therapy. This delivers oxygen through a tight fitting mask over the nose. The oxygen is pushed into lungs under gentle pressure, while the baby has to exhale on their own power."

"The lowest level of oxygen support is the nasal cannula. This uses a set of plastic prongs to deliver air into the nostrils. The baby has to use their own power to both inhale and exhale on this support level."

Modra goes on to explain each type of oxygen support has advantages—and disadvantages. Short-term oxygen gives the baby time to recover and build lung tissue; but long-term use actually harms the very tissue it is trying to save. Oxygen delivered by machine tends to open airways in the upper regions of the lungs—leaving the lower part of the lungs untouched and prone to collapse.

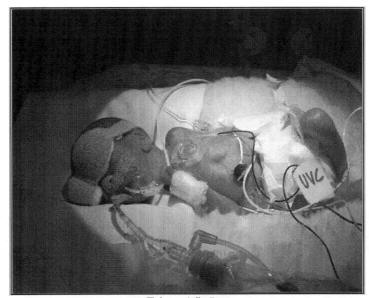

Ethan - 1 lb. 7 oz.

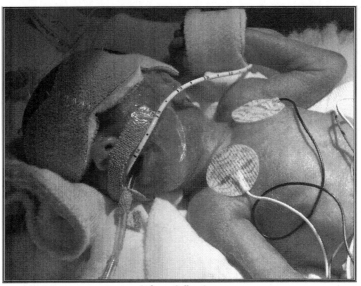

Aidan - 2 lbs. 1 oz.

Today Nurse Practitioner Josephine is on duty. Her long fuzzy bright red hair and delightful Australian accent are not the first things you notice; rather it is her great sense of humor. It's a rare gift she brings to a place that has so little to smile about.

Josephine's specialty is weaning babies from oscillating ventilators. Taking a seat next to me, she describes the process of carefully monitored steps used to move a baby off this machine. First, the shank mechanism will be turned off while Aidan is still hooked up to the oscillator. The shank causes the vibrations, which create puffs of air to keep the tiny under-developed lungs constantly inflated.

If Aidan handles the shank being turned off, she'll move to the next step of hooking up the ventilator. The oscillator will be left in place during the switchover as a precaution. If the lungs tolerate this and remain stable, Josephine will then disconnect the oscillator.

Each step is double and triple checked, and the process can take an entire afternoon to complete.

***

Oh no. Midway through weaning Aidan off the oscillator, his lungs hyper-extend. Aidan's systems become unstable as the oscillator over-inflates his lungs!

Josephine handles this situation with the calm nerves of a fighter pilot. She has to get Aidan off the oscillator as soon as possible. There's no time to complete all the weaning steps to the ventilator, so with a few quick moves she skillfully gets him onto CPAP oxygen support.

There is more bad news—Ethan can't be taken off the oscillator just yet—his stats are too unstable. Blood gas numbers show CO_2 levels have built up once again.

Josephine is giving Ethan a transfusion (*his seventh*). This is to improve the blood oxygen levels. Through all this Ethan needs to be kept calm—so she has him on fentanyl for pain management and as a sedative.

As the afternoon wears on, the stats continue to get worse. Ethan's glucose numbers are up to 359—well above the norm of 150. I am told elevated sugars can be a sign of infection. This has all of us very concerned.

***

By late afternoon Aidan's hyper-extended lungs are better, his blood gas reading has improved, and he is holding stable on CPAP. To be sure he has adequate oxygen saturation levels, Josephine is giving him another blood transfusion.

As the day winds down, I get more good news. Aidan is exhaling CO_2—all on his own!

Isn't this a strange update for a memory book? Other moms celebrate their baby's first coo or smile. I celebrate one of my sons can exhale.

The thought makes me want to cry.

***

At midnight Justin and I grab a cup of instant soup from the cafeteria vending machine. In the few minutes we were away, Ethan dislodged his oscillator tubing. All it takes is minuscule movement of the tube to move it from the optimum placement in the lungs.

Dr. Lesotho decides not to reinsert the tubing and places Ethan directly on CPAP—skipping the ventilator. He says this is not the ideal plan, but Ethan's throat is so swollen there is no way for him to get a vent tube inserted tonight.

Chapter 7 - *Aidan Cries, Ethan Crashes*

"On life's most difficult days
all that we can do is
simply take things moment by moment."

Kristi A. Dyer

Saturday, October 21, 2006
NICU Day 13

Our daily routine is for Justin and me to arrive at the hospital in time to hear early morning updates. Today however, Justin misses rounds—he's standing outside where his cell phone gets better reception. He is busy trying to preserve one of his business accounts. Justin and his partner run a small construction project management firm. It's such a struggle for him to run his company and be at the NICU every day. I can't imagine the stress he is dealing with as he watches our financial stability slip away as his company loses out in the bid process with more and more clients.

***

For the past 13 days our twins have been the only babies in the oversized Quad room, which is designed to hold four isolettes. The Admission office alerts the NICU staff that two more sets of twins are due to arrive at any time. They want us to move out of the Quad and into one of the smaller rooms designed to hold two isolettes. The nurse says the new room is quieter, has more subdued lighting, and there's a small sofa bench to sleep on. That's good news, as a bench means I have a place to actually lie down when I spend the night. No more trying to sleep propped upright in a chair.

The change in rooms is handled without a hitch. The boys' isolettes are wheeled down the short hall to a room that will be ours for the rest of the NICU stay. What we don't know at this time is the boys' journey through the NICU will last for more than *150 days*.

***

At midday rounds I meet another one of the NICU doctors—Dr. Baillie. I swear he looks like a twin of the Supreme Court Justice Clarence Thomas.

He works a few days each month in the NICU and the rest of his time he heads Mission Valley's Pediatric Clinic. That's a special clinic where fragile preemies' growth and development are monitored after they are discharged from the hospital.

As we wait a short minute or two for the other doctors to join rounds, one of the nurses takes this time to explain the purpose of the outpatient clinic.

"After discharge from the NICU, extremely premature babies need ongoing treatment for five to seven years. That's the optimum window of time to resolve health and development issues."

I want to view this in a positive light. We have five years (*I refuse to think in terms of a seven-year sentence*) to resolve health issues and put this all behind us. Naïve to be sure, but I don't care. I will get my babies home and begin the five-year count down. A simple enough strategy, but I don't fool myself into really believing this. I can't think more than a day—or an hour—into the future.

The rest of the doctors arrive for rounds and Dr. Baillie begins the update. "Ethan had several apnea[17] episodes last night and gave everyone a hard time by not regulating his breathing."

He looks down at his notes for a moment, and then says to me; "This is not unusual. Preemies generally have this problem starting in the first week or so of life. We can treat apnea with medication if this gets severe enough. For now, this is not a major deal. We'll just keep on eye on it."

---

[17]Apnea is a precipitous drop in respirations. During an apnea spell, a baby stops breathing for 20 seconds or longer, the heart rate may decrease, and the skin may turn pale or blue. Apnea is usually caused by immaturity in the area of the brain that controls the drive to breathe.

We all stand in a circle around Ethan's isolette as Dr. Baillie continues his update. Suddenly, I am aware of a strange mewing sound coming from the direction of Aidan's isolette.

Oh my gosh! *I can hear Aidan crying.*

Without the ventilator tube down his throat, I can finally hear Aidan. His cry sounds like a newborn kitten. So faint and nearly silent—but I hear it.

To my surprise, his cry makes my milk let down and my clothes are quickly soaked with breast milk.

As I pull on a sweater to hide my wet shirt, I see one of the nurses is giving Aidan a teeny tiny pacifier about an inch long. He does not have the strength to latch on and the pacifier readily falls from his mouth.

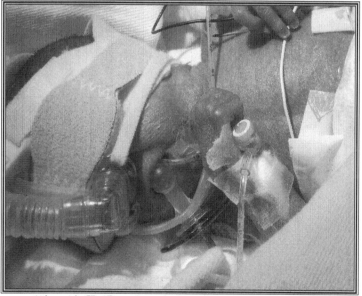

Aidan with CPAP mask, eyeshades, and a one-inch long mini pacifier

***

Crisis again! In one short hour, we've gone from joy to despair. Ethan is crashing. He was moved too fast from the full breathing support of the oscillator all the way down to

CPAP. At first it looked like he was adjusting to the lower support, but after a few hours we're losing ground. His lungs are not strong enough. It took his entire reserve of strength just to exhale CO_2 from his lungs. He has nothing left to give. He cannot exhale anymore.

Dr. Lim warned the medical team to keep Ethan on the oscillator and not to move him to CPAP too soon. Just because Ethan had a good few hours, it does not mean his lungs are strong enough to exhale on his own. It's like forcing Ethan to run a marathon. He can't keep up this pace.

I wish they had been able to reinsert the vent tube last night. Have we lost precious lung tissue with this fiasco?

To complicate things, Ethan is down to only two viable IV spots. All the rest of his IVs have blown. And, as if to pile on more bad news, the lab cultures are back. The results confirm Ethan has an infection.

I have a sinking feeling about this.

Sunday, October 22, 2006
NICU Day 14

than is crying silently. This breaks my heart. I want to hold and comfort my son, but he can't be held. In fact, I can't get any closer to Ethan than the armholes cut in the side of his isolette.

I try to find an area of skin on Ethan to touch and to soothe him. But it seems that every inch of his body is covered with IVs, tubes and monitor wires. My hand is so big it could cover him like a blanket.

When Ethan clasps hold of my finger, I feel an immense wave of helplessness. I know this struggle for survival has to be fought by one so small. All of us here at the hospital are his helpers—but the one that has to win this battle is Ethan.

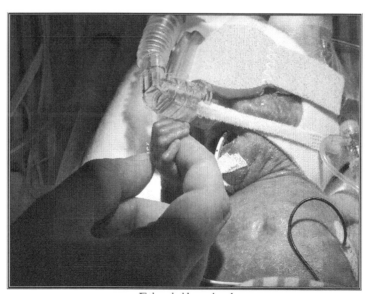

Ethan holds my hand

***

The nurse weighs Ethan using a scale built into the isolette. He's holding steady at 660 grams today—about 14 grams less than his birth weight.

She looks up at me and says in a near whisper; "You know, Ethan is the smallest surviving preemie ever at Mission Valley. He's our miracle baby."

I don't like the moniker 'miracle baby' as it does not seem to give credit to the Herculean efforts of the medical team—nor to the boys themselves as they fight the issues of extreme prematurity. And I don't like the term because it sounds passive—as if we are dependent on the spin of a dial. Maybe you win a miracle and maybe you don't.

I prefer to call my boys 'dragon tamers'. They are fighting hard to tame the dragons of prematurity not to bite.

Deep in my soul, however, I know it will take a miracle to win this fight.

Monday, October 23, 2006
NICU Day 15

arly this morning Justin and I talk about finances. It's just him and his business partner running the company. We're going to flounder if Justin doesn't get his business back on solid footing. If his company fails, we have no income.

We've come to a decision. Justin will focus his energy on reviving his business accounts and I'll be at the hospital every day.

I make the long drive to the NICU alone this morning, knowing if the situation is urgent I can call Justin to come quickly. Of course I am not really alone; Nana and Papa are here with me. They will come to the hospital every day until this nightmare is over. My family is like the shore where I tether my boat—solid and always there for me.

***

Dr. Baillie stops by with an update on Aidan's brain scan. He is wearing a huge smile—so I know the results even before he speaks.

"Aidan's x-ray shows no more hyper-extension in his lungs and the heart echocardiogram shows the PDA hole has stayed closed. I think I can even decrease his CPAP by a full setting today."

The doctor pulls up a wheeled stool and sits down to give the rest of his update. As he leans over Aidan's isolette, my son opens both eyes wide and *smiles*.

"Look," I said, "Aidan is smiling!"

Papa is perched on the stool next to Ethan's isolette and says with a laugh, "It's probably just gas!"

"Ha! How can you know gas from a smile? I *know* Aidan smiled at me," I tease back.

Our lighthearted banter is dampened when Dr. Baillie shifts his weight on the stool and clears his throat.

I sense he is about to give bad news.

The doctor leans forward and rests his elbows on his knees. Drawing in a deep breath he says, "The blood clot from Ethan's Stage II brain bleed has moved. The clot is now plugging the hole where brain fluid drains from the ventricles. This in turn causes fluid to build up and swell, and the swelling presses on Ethan's brain tissue."

I'm looking at Dr. Baillie and I am sure he thinks I am taking this in—but my mind is shutting down. I am trying to understand his words, but the only thing my brain registers is that his lips are moving. I may look as if I am engaged in this discussion, but stress dampens all sound.

Thank goodness Nana and Papa are here. Nana takes copious notes and asks all the right questions as Dr. Baillie goes on to explain this might be a serious problem. He'll wait until Monday to do another brain scan. Maybe we'll see the clot resolve itself—or maybe it will move and cause more swelling elsewhere in the brain.

Oh how I hate Mondays. It seems every Monday brings bad news.

Chapter 8 - *A Gift of Hope*

"Just as despair can come to one another only
from other human beings,
hope too, can be given to one only
by another human being."

Elie Wiesel

Tuesday, October 24, 2006
NICU Day 16

E than opened his eyes! Well, one eye anyway—the right eye is still fused closed. He gets his first look at the world and *it's a plastic box!* I wonder what he thinks about all of this. I tell him not to judge things too harshly. There is more to life than this.

***

Since birth, Aidan and Ethan's nutrition has been supplied by something called Total Parenteral Nutrition—or TPN for short. This is made up of the most basic pre-digested components of nutrition. It's given by way of an IV directly into the circulatory system since the baby's intestines are not yet mature enough to breakdown food.

It can be disastrous if an unstable preemie is given food too soon. It can cause problems such as NEC[18]—a dreadful condition where the intestines become infected and tissue dies. This disabling condition can even be life threatening.

Ethan is too unstable to consider breast milk, but Aidan may be ready in a week or so. When he gets his first breast milk, it will be mixed with additives and fed into his stomach through a nasogastric (NG) feeding tube.

I am glad at least one of my boys will be ready for breast milk, as I've been up around the clock pumping

---

[18] Necrotizing enterocolitis (NEC) is an infection of the intestine in premature babies after they have begun feeding. At birth, the baby's gastrointestinal track contains no bacteria. Once feeding begins, the normal process of bacteria colonization of the intestine begins. In premature babies, their immature immune system is not ready for this process and infection may occur. In severe cases of NEC, surgery may be required to remove sections of the intestines. Symptoms can come on rapidly and in extreme cases NEC can be fatal.

every three hours since they were born. I feel like a prize milk cow.

To help keep things lighthearted, Nana hung a tiny wooden cow on my breast-pump bag. Even Dr. Placket laughs and says he personally holds me responsible for filling the NICU freezer to capacity with breast milk.

We hope once the boys are able to take milk they will put on weight. Nana creates a chart for our journal where I can post the boys' daily weight. Much to the medical teams' chagrin, I begin an obsessive check every day for weight changes. It is a tangible thing I can relate to and it helps me to see progress—or lack of.

Each morning Nana and I greet the nurses with, "How many grams today?"

Anticipating our needs, the nursing staff posts the daily weights on the room white-board. One of the nurses even draws a cute cartoon on the board to celebrate days when the boys have a weight gain. Besides the hand-colored nametags hanging above their isolettes, the cartoon doodles are the only festive decorations in the room.

***

The medical team gathers in the boys' room, as afternoon rounds are about to start. Dr. Placket leads off with a review of the twin's current stats; then shifts to potential long-term outcomes.

"Four milestones are typically used to predict the prognosis of a preemie in the first seven days of life—but for a *micro-preemie,*" he says with added emphasis, "there is one more hurdle to meet. If a micro-preemie can make it to the two-week mark, be stable and not have any new illnesses, the odds increase in their favor. If a baby makes it this far the survival rate goes up."

While he tries to keep a non-committal expression on his face, I can see a smile form in his expressive eyes as he continues.

"Ethan's initial chances of survival were less than 20% because he had three strikes against him. First, he is very small. Second, he has the worst lung problems I've ever seen in a preemie; and third, he has a brain hemorrhage."

"These are three strikes, but Ethan is not out. And as long as both boys don't develop new health issues—the ones they have now are survivable."

This is the first time we hear the word *survivable*. I fixate on the word and for once I breathe without anxiety chest pains.

With this one word, Dr. Placket gives me what I so desperately wanted—*hope*. I could have kissed him.

I know he is not making a promise of survival—but hope turns our whole world around. Parents' should always have hope for their children's future.

Wednesday, October 25, 2006
NICU Day 17

Nurse Practitioner Josephine was on rotation a week ago. I am glad to see that she is back again today.

As she tucks a stray strand of curly red hair underneath her scrub cap, Josephine says, "I am so surprised at how well the boys are doing. These guys are real fighters. A week ago I didn't give them much of a chance."

I know Josephine means this as a compliment on the boys' remarkable progress. I am so proud of my sons for fighting hard to survive these past 17 days.

Josephine is in charge of rounds this morning. She starts the debriefing off with an update of Aidan's stats.

"His blood gas is good this morning, however he did not tolerate CPAP being turned down a full notch—so I pushed this up to a setting of 6.0 for now. We'll give Aidan his first breast milk today. We'll only give him a very small amount to be sure his intestines are working properly."

The update continues as Josephine moves next to Ethan's stats.

"Of course, there's no plan to give Ethan breast milk. He is still too unstable to risk giving him food. He'll stay on the TPN for now. His blood gas is not doing well. It shows acidosis—this is a serious situation that weakens all of the body systems."

Glancing down at her notes Josephine concludes; "His glucose level is way too high. There is a lot to deal with here, and we have this little guy on a serious regiment of meds to handle these latest issues."

I ask for an update on the oxygen support.

"In the ongoing effort to wean Ethan off the vent, he has been shifted back and forth from ventilator to CPAP and back again several times. I'm sorry—we just can't find a stable baseline for this baby."

Unstable seems to sum it up.

I am trying so hard not to jump to the worst-case scenario. When the last of the medical team leaves the room, I take a highlighter pen to underline any positive words in today's notes. I just can't find any for Ethan.

***

It has been a long day. Nana and I gather up our jackets and cell phones and head to the parking lot. On the way out, we pause to say good night to Lacy at the NICU front desk. I notice a large vase of colorful flowers on the counter. This bright summer bouquet seems a bit out of place for a cold and rainy October.

Propped in front of the vase is a note card. My eyes scan the card, but I quickly look away before reading any more. The first line says, "In remembrance of Baby Allen…"

The flowers are from the family of the baby who was in the room next to ours—a room now silent.

I say a prayer for this family that left the NICU empty handed.

Thursday, October 26, 2006
NICU Day 18

Coming onto the NICU floor early this morning, I glance down the long hallway to my babies' room. Dr. Placket is sitting there all alone with the lights off. He is perched on a high stool with one arm slung over the top of Ethan's isolette. This gives me such a scare my legs can hardly carry me down the hallway.

As I rush into the room, Dr. Placket looks up.

"Not to worry," he says quickly. "Everything is fine now. I'm just having quiet time with Ethan."

As he debriefs me however, I find out it was a long night of unstable stats. My baby was so agitated they had to give him morphine. Even with this strong drug, Dr. Placket had to take Ethan off CPAP and put him back on the ventilator.

"We won't try to wean Ethan off the vent for another two weeks. I had a heck of a time getting the vent tube in. Ethan's larynx is so swollen the tube was nearly impossible to insert."

While one of the nurses hooks Ethan up to yet another blood transfusion (*his ninth*), Dr. Placket continues the debriefing.

"Ethan's lungs are much more fragile than first indicated. This little guy needs to gain 200 grams before we can reconsider taking him off the vent. I am afraid he just does not have enough chest muscle to exhale."

***

By mid morning Ethan's ventilator tube has dislodged again. The smallest movement of just a half-inch can shift it from the optimal placement spot inside his lungs. When this happens, the doctor has to pull the tube out entirely and start over. This is now two times in one day! Ethan's throat is terribly swollen and reinserting vent tubes is certainly not helping matters. I wonder why they can't do something to keep the tube in place so it won't dislodge so easily.

By 2:00 PM Ethan's ventilator tube has been dislodged *twice more.* Now we are up to four times in one day. I am incensed! Come on people! This team needs to find a better way to prevent this.

I feel the tension in the room until Dr. Placket lightens the mood. "For a 680 gram baby to dislodge his tube four times in one day," he says, "means he's not very sick!"

Of course, we all know this is NICU humor. I can tell Dr. Placket is exasperated having to intubate this baby again and again.

***

People don't know what to say to a new mom and dad of critically ill babies. They say the wrong things, not out of malice but from a lack of understanding.

One of my neighbors stops by to give us a dinner casserole. She babbles on that she had also planned to give us a gift of matching baby outfits—but took the clothes back to the store because she didn't think the boys would survive and only had 30 days to get a full refund.

Seeing my face fall in shock, she says, "Don't worry Honey. If they survive, of course I'll buy them a new outfit!"

***

New to me are feelings of complete vulnerability. Anything will set me off—even a kind word from a stranger asking, 'How are you today?'

I am fighting back tears and the ache in my chest is ever-present. It keeps me awake at night. I try to sleep, but my heart is stretched so thin I think it might burst.

The nights are the most difficult. All my feelings come alive and this is the time I feel more adrift and lost than any other part of my day.

Chapter 9 - *Kanga Holds Roo*

"Making a decision to have a child—it's momentous.
It is to decide forever to have
your heart go walking outside your body."

Elizabeth Stone

Friday October 27, 2006
NICU Day 19

It's a good-news day when the nurse tells me *I can hold Aidan!* My son is 19 days old and I get to hold him for the very first time.

I am so excited I telephone Nana. "You'll want to leave work early today to come see the babies—and bring the camera!"

Next, I speed dial Justin and leave a voice message. "Your son has a surprise to show you this afternoon!"

The sun is shining—today is going to be a good day.

***

Nurse Angelica stops by to chat. She's tall and graceful as a dancer, with gorgeous long dark hair softly pulled back off her face. She was the night-shift nurse assigned to Ethan on the day he was born.

"I am so pleased to see how well they are doing," she says. "You know everyone in the medical community is following the boys' progress on your *CarePage* website."

Flashing a shy smile she adds; "They made quite a stir being the tiniest ever at the hospital—even our hospital's CEO stops in to see them every now and then."

I think to myself the CEO probably wants to see the million dollar babies. But really, I know he too must care about these tiny twins. I am just blown away by compassion of everyone at this hospital.

***

I run into Dr. Placket at the NICU admin desk, where he sits reading medical records on the computer.

"How did the morning lab work turn out for Aidan's bloody stool?" I ask.

"Just now looking this up. Would you like to look with me?"

As I look over Dr. Placket's shoulder at the computer monitor, he reads the lab report aloud and interprets the results into layman's terms.

"Aidan's bowel movement tested positive for blood; however, the scan results of his intestines look fine to me. There's no indication as to why blood was in the stool. It might just be an odd coincidence—or it might be a sign that the intestines are not tolerating breast milk."

"For now, I am taking Aidan off breast milk and we'll continue to monitor for blood in the stool. If it's warranted, a full set of abdominal x-rays will be ordered to make sure this is not the beginning signs of NEC."

In my readings on preemie health issues, I learned about the dreaded NEC, so I don't ask Dr. Placket any more questions. I already know how serious NEC is for a fragile preemie.

Dr. Placket taught me—way back in the first days of this NICU journey—to take medical issues as they come and not borrow troubles from tomorrow. So I decide not to worry about NEC for now.

I leave Dr. Placket at the Nurses' Station where he continues to read the rest of the twin's lab results and head down the hall to the boys' room.

Nurses Angelica and Modra are waiting for me in the doorway. They are literally bouncing on their toes and brimming over with good news.

They burst out in unison; "Ethan's brain scan shows no additional bleeding—the swelling is going down!"

The nurses were reading the lab updates on the computer in the boys' room. It's an unofficial update of course, as they are supposed to wait for the doctor to complete his reading—but the news is so good they can't wait to spill the beans.

I pretend not to know this as Dr. Placket enters the room wearing a big grin. I want him to be able to tell me the news himself.

Dr. Placket winks towards Angelica and Modra as he tells me, "I am pleased to be able to give you good news today—for once without being preempted by the nurses."

We just grin and keep our secret; however I think he already knows the nurses beat him to it.

***

The day continues with more reasons to smile. Today I get to hold my son.

Picking up a one pound baby to cuddle takes planning. The hold, called a *kangaroo hold*, is where baby and mom are bare skin-to-skin. It's comforting for a baby to hear his mama's heartbeat and cuddle against her warm skin.

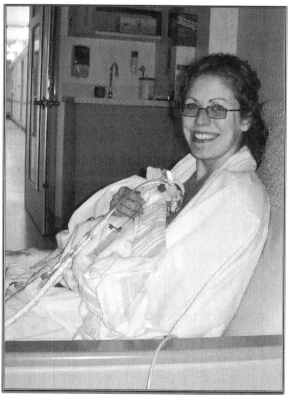

Look close... I am holding Aidan for the first time!

I'm excited, but a bit puzzled. How can I hold Aidan with all the monitor wires, IVs, and CPAP paraphernalia?

Once we figure it out and Aidan is snug in my arms, all the wires and tubes seem to disappear.

It's difficult to hold back the tears as I cuddle with my darling son. There were so many times I thought I would never be able to hold him.

Nana is busy taking photos and Justin leans over my shoulder talking to Aidan. I know I should offer Justin a chance to hold his son as well, but I refuse to let go.

While I sit with Aidan, one of the doctors stops by to tell me Ethan's new arterial line is not working correctly. They may have to take it out after the next blood gas reading if they can't get a good draw through the line.

He also notes Ethan is very agitated and they had to give him another dose of morphine to help him sleep. The remaining tests for today are cancelled to let Ethan rest and stabilize.

It has been a long and eventful day. I am still on an emotional high from holding Aidan. As Justin and I prepare to leave, I lean over each isolette and tell my sons, "Goodnight—I'll see you in the morning."

We make the 45-minute drive home, attend to the pets, throw a load of clothes in the washer, and crawl into bed.

Justin is asleep as soon as his head hits the pillow.

Reaching for the phone, I place a call to the NICU for one more status update on the twins. Dr. Lesotho is on duty this evening. The news he has to deliver is unsettling.

"I am having hard time with your baby's blood pressure. I do not know what is causing pressure to drop," he says in his clipped accent.

"And I give to your baby much morphine as sedative and much dopamine to raise blood pressure. Please. Know this. Your baby remains unstable."

I know which twin the doctor is talking about without him ever saying Ethan's name aloud.

This leaves me frozen with indecision.

Should I go to the hospital now or wait till morning?

Hearing Justin snore as he falls into deep slumber, I decide to wait; I don't want to wake him.

I just lie here unable to sleep as my thoughts whirl in a vicious circle of dreadful worries.

Saturday, October 28, 2006
NICU Day 20

E than had a rough night and his blood pressure instability continues this morning. He is on dopamine and morphine, but even with all this medication his respirator alarm keeps going off.

The doctors are not entirely sure why. Dr. Placket tells me this might be because the swelling in Ethan's throat is going down and the ventilator tube is moving around in his trachea—allowing air to back-wash out of his throat. Each time air backwashes, the alarms go off. However, Dr. Lesotho disagrees. He thinks the blood pressure instability is because of an open PDA.

***

By afternoon some of our stress is lifted. It's funny how our spirits drop and soar in the span of just an hour. This afternoon vitals are stable for both boys. This lifts the ever-present fog of stress and we try to lighten the mood by giving Aidan a nickname. We call him 'Snorkel Bob' because the CPAP mask and coiled tubing looks a bit like snorkel gear.

Even with all the stress, the NICU has its own dark brand of humor. Ethan is the comedy act today. He has a small Velcro patch on his scalp holding an IV in place and on his left hand is another IV wrapped in Velcro. When he jerks his left arm, it flops up and lands on his temple—sticking fast to the Velcro on the scalp! With his left arm stuck to his forehead, he jerks his right arm as if to get out of this predicament—and his right arm sticks fast to the scalp Velcro too! Now both arms are stuck crossed over his forehead. I should take a picture, but I am laughing too hard as I reach through the armholes in the side of the isolette to gently rescue my little comedian.

Sunday, October 29, 2006
NICU Day 21

Aidan weighs nearly two pounds. Nurse Julie tells me much of this weight is because of the multiple blood transfusions he got this morning.

Dr. Lesotho stops by and immediately frowns as he leans over Aidan's isolette.

"I see this baby is moved to the cannula. I do not like cannula used with babies this small. They do not have chest muscle to exhale. At first sign of difficulty I will put Aidan back to CPAP. You understand? Yes?"

He continues his staccato stream of comments without pausing. "Aidan has blood in his stool again. This can be because of trauma of NG tube in the stomach; reaction to high dose of hydrocortisone; open PDA valve; or beginning of NEC."

Damn. So do you have any more bad news for me?

Did I say this aloud? I was just thinking this—but I sense Dr. Lesotho read my mind as he arches his eyebrows at me.

He flashes a tight-lipped smile that seems to be his telltale sign for bad news.

"I heard heart murmur in Aidan today. This can mean the PDA valve re-opened. I scheduled heart scan for Monday to confirm. If PDA is opened slightly, it will probably close again on its own. If fully open, you need to take this baby for surgery."

He turns and sweeps his arm in the direction of Ethan's isolette. "Your other baby's PDA may have reopened too. This boy has all the signs of wide-open PDA. I called for a scan for this baby on Monday as well."

I still hate Mondays.

Morning rounds are ready to start. The rest of the doctors and nurses have streamed into the boys' room. As each one gives their update, I scribble notes into my journal.

The nurse says Ethan's weight is 710 grams (~1 lb. 9 oz.) and his stats fluctuated last night. His blood pressure is now holding at 27.

Dr. Lesotho brusquely interrupts the nurse's update. "Low blood pressure should be treated with dopamine. And I believe this baby may need PDA surgery."

Raising his head and looking directly at me, Dr. Placket calmly counters this view explaining blood pressure of 27 is borderline and that it is best not to chase Ethan's vitals up and down the scale with meds. Glancing over at Dr. Lesotho, he adds firmly; "And I feel it is premature to suggest surgery at this point."

The two doctors disagree and Dr. Placket concludes rounds saying he will contact a sub-specialist for insight on treating fluctuating blood pressure in babies with as many issues as Ethan.

However, as the medical team breaks from rounds, I hear Dr. Lesotho give an order to the last nurse leaving the room to put Ethan on dopamine.

***

At noon Dr. Lesotho places an order for Ethan to be given breast milk. Have things improved that much? Just this morning he was disagreeing on the treatment of Ethan's blood pressure. Since milk can't be given to an unstable baby without risking a trigger for NEC, I figure Ethan's pressure must have stabilized. In hindsight, I ought to have questioned this.

After the midday rounds, I notice Dr. Lesotho at the end of the long hallway talking with my visiting in-laws. The words of their conversation carry clearly over the background noise of the NICU.

"This baby could have more problems with brain bleeds," he tells them. "The real statistic you should have as your priority is not ventilation issues. Rather you should be concerned with head circumference reading. Any change in the circumference is how we judge severity of brain bleeds."

He stresses with my in-laws; "It is time for you to take charge. These babies must be moved to Mercy Hospital. You must turn their care over to sub-specialists. You understand? Yes?"

My in-laws agree with Dr. Lesotho and in turn lobby Justin and me to force a transfer of our sons to Mercy.

The stress this division brings to our family is unbelievable. The situation we're in is hard enough without this extra drama.

I wish I had taken the time earlier to talk with Dr. Lesotho about his lobby efforts. I let this go on far too long—I don't see how I can stop it now.

It is clear doctors can view the same set of medical facts and come to different opinions. I'm okay with this; but when they disagree on treatment plans, this is to be addressed only with the parents. It is not okay to lobby other family members to veto the parents' decision.

Chapter 10 - *Flatline*

"Anyone can give up; it's the easiest thing in the world to do.
But to hold it together when everyone else
would understand if you fell apart,
that's true strength."

Unknown

Crisis! Dr. Lesotho says he almost lost Ethan. In the early morning hours Ethan had a massive drop in blood pressure and his heart stopped.

I glare with disbelief into Dr. Lesotho's eyes as he says, "I had to give your baby chest compressions to revive him."

He tells me this as if reciting dull facts; however his voice trembles as he recalls the emotion of the near fatal night.

I'll be forever grateful for his skilled efforts that saved my precious Ethan—but I want to know why did this happen? And why the hell wasn't I called?

It is surreal to be told your baby's heart stopped and had chest compressions to save his life. How am I supposed to digest this information? Do I scream in anger or cry in fear? I do neither. I go into autopilot and robotically ask the doctor to explain what happened and what is in store next.

***

Dr. Lim stops by the room early this morning to tell me Ethan's blood pressure is still too low. Maybe the PDA is open again; but he doesn't think this caused the massive pressure drop that triggered the cardiopulmonary arrest last night. He thinks the drop is most likely due to infection.

Ethan's lungs are full of inflammation and they need to rule out infection; however high doses of steroids can mask the presence of bacteria making lab work inconclusive.

I switch gears and ask Dr. Lim about yesterday's order to give Ethan breast milk. Could that be part of the problem?

Dr. Lim is surprised to hear an order was made for breast milk. He comments that Ethan has too many vitals that are not yet stable.

"It is unwise to introduce breast milk at the same time blood pressure is unstable," he says. "Milk given to a baby with unstable blood pressure or with inflamed lungs can trigger NEC, and NEC is more prevalent in low birth weight kids. This presents a *triple concern* for Ethan."

***

As the doctors gather in the boys' room for afternoon rounds, I hear Dr. Lesotho say a heart scan must be ordered right away to rule out an open PDA.

Dr. Lim counters that he is more interested in getting the lab work re-done to verify if an infection is brewing.

"I'll look at the heart scan," Dr. Lim says, "but I am doubtful the PDA is causing this problem. I really think this is because of an infection. I am puzzled as to why the lab tests continue to be negative. With all the symptoms, this has to be because of infection."

The rounds seem to be at an impasse. The doctors have differing views on priorities—one sees PDA as the primary focus and one sees a brewing infection as primary.

Dr. Lesotho delivers a sharply worded counter opinion. "In my experience this baby must be sent for PDA surgery as soon as possible. You must do this."

The conversation stops. I hold my breath and watch the doctors closely. No one says anything for several seconds.

Dr. Lim breaks the silence when he calmly, and with much simplicity, counters with a single word; "No."

He continues his debriefing. "Ethan is on the highest dose of dopamine we can give and his blood pressure finally went back up. Something happened this weekend to make the blood pressure unstable. While the inconclusive lab work makes this a challenge to decipher, I wonder if

Ethan's heavy doses of steroids have made it hard for the lab to identify infection."

Dr. Lim muses aloud. "This could also be due to a problem with the adrenal glands—which regulate blood pressure. They may have burned out so to speak." He quickly shakes his head, as if to dismiss his own idea.

He repeats his biggest worry is Ethan has an infection.

"I am considering whether to give steroids again, as these worked well in the past—but I really don't want to use steroids as these can mask the real cause of the low blood pressure."

Turning to me, Dr. Lim says ever so gently, "If this is an infection, babies this size can go down fast."

***

By late afternoon Dr. Lesotho comes alone to find me in the boys' room.

With his heavy accent he says, "Heart scan shows wide-open PDA in both of your babies. Surgery is in order. Now is time to transfer these babies for surgery. Yes?"

Ignoring this, I excuse myself to go find a cup of coffee. While on the pretend-hunt for coffee, I once again go looking for the other doctors to ask if surgery is a consensus decision.

I find Dr. Lim entering data at the computer station. He abruptly stops mid-task with my interruption and rests his hands on his lap.

Giving me his full attention he calmly replies, "No surgery is warranted. Aidan's stats are doing well and we need to leave the PDA alone for now. Surgical intervention for Aidan would have a negative effect. I will re-evaluate this decision if he needs more breathing support in the future."

"As for Ethan," Dr. Lim adds gently, "this little one is so unstable the word *surgery* can't even be used in the same sentence as Ethan's name."

***

It's just an hour later and bad news piles on.

Dr. Lim has come to tell me the latest brain scan shows Ethan's brain bleed—originally described as a mild Grade II—has now increased to somewhere between a Grade II and a Grade III.

I can't breathe and I don't move. My body is locked rigid as all my senses strain to understand what he is telling me.

"The right side is where the original brain bleed occurred," he explains. "The right ventricle is larger than the left. Debris has blocked the ventricle hole where fluid is supposed to drain. The fluid is accumulating and causing swelling. You may hear other doctors use the term *hydrocephalus* to describe this condition."

Dr. Lim pauses a moment, then continues. "This is not unexpected and we will watch this closely. The plan is to measure Ethan's head circumference daily and do an ultrasound every week to monitor the situation."

To soften the blow, he empathetically adds; "Ethan does not have a full Grade III bleed. He is somewhere in-between a Grade II and a Grade III."

With his words carefully wrapped in a thin tissue of hope, Dr. Lim explains further. "Assigning grades to measure brain bleeds was done long before today's technology. We can now measure bleeding in the brain with much more finite accuracy. There are a wide range of issues within each grade, so the impact is not as black and white as the assignment of Grade II or Grade III might imply."

***

It has been a long day of failing stats. Ethan's blood pressure should be in the target range of 32 to 38—but it continues to be in the low 20's.

He is so lethargic I can barely see any sign of life.

The lab results are still inconclusive. Even so, Dr. Lim did not wait on them—he began to treat Ethan for a suspected infection many hours earlier.

Dr. Lim is convinced there is a bacterium present. He orders the lab to re-run all the blood cultures once more. Without a firm identification of *which type* of bacteria strain is present, it is hard adjust a proper mix of antibiotics.

***

Just when you think it can't get any worse, it does.

By late evening the lab work is back and it shows Ethan has sepsis—a life threatening infection that has spread into his circulatory system.

I remember Dr. Lim's earlier words; "*...with infections, babies this small can go down fast...*"

The lab confirms the infection is caused by a Gram-negative bacterium called *Serratia*. The doctor suspects the infection entered the blood stream via one of Ethan's many IV sites. The bacterium is rampant throughout Ethan's body and exploded into a condition called Disseminated Intravascular Coagulation[19]; or as it is more commonly known, DIC.

---

[19] Disseminated Intravascular Coagulation (DIC)—definition source: Michele Kemper's lecture notes [San Jose State University; *Morbidity of the Neonate*, circa 1973; professor's name long forgotten.]

DIC is associated with a poor prognosis and a high mortality rate. It readily occurs in NICU patients with extensive trauma—especially those with Gram-negative sepsis. DIC is a process where the blood starts to coagulate throughout the body. One critical aspect of DIC is the release of a glycoprotein called Tissue Factor (TF). As TF is circulated, it activates the coagulation cascade. In short, the blood cells disintegrate and leave multiple clots in the circulation. These excess clots trap platelets to become larger clots, which leads to thrombosis and paradoxically an increased risk of hemorrhage. The lodging of clots throughout the circulatory system and internal organs leads to organ degeneration, shock, and hypotension. Prognosis for low-birth weight babies is poor with a high mortality rate.

Nana recalls what this means in terms of a prognosis from her university studies so many years earlier. However, she keeps these details to herself. All she shares with me is; "This will be a tough fight."

I know this is a dreadful condition.

I don't ask questions.

I don't want to hear the answer.

Chapter 11 - *Edge of Survival*

"In all things it is better to hope than to despair."

Johann Wolfgang van Goethe

Today is Halloween. The leaves have blown off the trees and the weather has turned cold and damp. Here in the NICU it is a constant 72°—as if there are no seasons and no march of time.

Some of the staff dress in costume and the hallways are lined with fall decorations.

It is hard to imagine life going on outside the hospital. I feel like there are no holidays, no celebrations, and no normalcy. I do not watch the news. I do not care what is happening at work. I rarely laugh. Nothing can bring me happiness until I know my sons will survive.

When we are invited to a Halloween party, I beg off saying we need to stay close by the babies.

"Why can't you come?" our hosts respond. "The NICU is like having a free baby-sitter!"

These people are so far removed from our nightmare world. I can't even talk with them on the same level any more.

***

Ethan received more platelets and three more blood transfusions this morning. The transfusions are helping to flush out the DIC and replace dead blood cells with fresh ones.

As blood is fed into Ethan's IV, I stare at his translucent skin and swear I can see inside his veins where blood cells are rushing off to fight this massive infection. I sit transfixed—as if my mind alone has the strength to will these blood cells to win the fight.

Ethan is so fragile; his health issues have more dramatic ups and downs. Hour-by-hour, minute-by-minute, we watch as he lurches between stable and unstable.

The blood transfusions are not working—in fact his blood cells are continuing to die off at an alarmingly fast rate and fill his veins with blood clots. Ethan's lungs are so cloudy and his respirations are severely labored.

The doctors seem to be in a perpetual huddle of conferences as they try to solve the mystery of Ethan's multi-layered symptoms.

The medical team is preparing me for the worst. In careful words they let it be known Ethan is at the edge of survival.

My senses are so wounded I labor to breathe. My brain feels sluggish and thinking is locked into repetitive circles.

***

Ethan has been on a cocktail of antibiotics for 24 hours. By late afternoon his blood pressure shows signs of improving.

Dare I hope?

Dr. Placket stops by the room. He has a three-day growth of beard and his scrubs look like he slept in them. Just as he enters the room, Ethan starts to act fussy and more like his normal agitated self.

The doctor's eyes look tired, but he smiles with his whole face.

"Seeing Ethan fussy makes me feel relieved and positive again," he says.

As the doctor leaves the room, Nurse Modra casually mentions aloud to no one in particular; "Dr. Placket has been here 72 hours straight—polling every specialist there is on this case. If anyone can figure this out, he will."

Wednesday, November 1, 2006
NICU Day 24

Aidan has gained weight! The nurse says he is now a whooping 964 grams (~2 lbs. 2 oz.). My new nickname for him is Chunky Monkey. Bet no one has ever called a two-pound baby Chunky!

Hitting the two-pound mark is a relief. We view this milestone as meaning we won't have to worry *every day* about Aidan's survival. As NICU parents we make-up events to celebrate—normal baby books just don't cover this experience.

***

While Aidan has the good-news of weight gain, it's another day of bad news for Ethan.

Dr. Lim tells us the infection has not been stopped—it spread throughout the entire circulatory system. Ethan is receiving cryoprecipitate, platelets, and another blood transfusion (*his 14th*). If they can get the infection under control, the expectation is the blood coagulation from DIC will correct itself. In the meantime, multiple blood transfusions are to help keep him alive.

This is a critical setback, yet Dr. Lim softens the blow with a series of positives before ending on a cautionary note.

"The treatment for infection is starting to take hold. The adrenal glands are working. Blood pressure looks okay for now, and the electrolyte balance is getting better. We are pointed away from the edge; but Ethan is far from stable."

***

Being on the brink of death so many times is taking its toll on the family. Stress does funny things—we develop selective hearing. Today, in the midst of the dire update on the spreading DIC crisis, we listen for any thing sounding positive. When we hear *"...the lungs are looking better,"* we take these words out of context and ignore the part that says Ethan is still unable breathe on his own. We take apart these medical updates bit by bit until we find a shred of good news.

We know this is unrealistic, but we're on the cliff ready to tip over at any moment. Trust me. *We know.*

Nana and I are unusually quiet at rounds today. I don't like the doctors searching my face to see if I understand how dire this is. I don't want to hear the words. Not today.

Deep in my soul I know Ethan is leaving us.

Damn it; don't make me acknowledge it aloud.

***

The stress is weighing me down. I am prone to tears and unable to sleep. I have no appetite and have massive anxiety attacks. I hold it together at the hospital and fall apart as soon as I leave. My routine is to cry throughout the entire drive to and from the hospital in the privacy of my car.

I failed to hold on to my pregnancy until my babies' due date.

What went so terribly wrong?

Chapter 12 - *Whiteout*

When the world says, "Give up"
Hope whispers, "Try one more time."

Unknown

Thursday, November 2, 2006
NICU Day 25

There are two stories today for the journal. One is of great joy watching Aidan grow stronger. The other is of despair, as Ethan seems to be leaving us.

***

I get another kangaroo hold with Aidan. As I hold him in my arms, my two-pound baby tries to turn his own head—but he can't. All the CPAP gear on his face makes this impossible. I have to help Aidan with this simple task of turning his head.

There is a light tickle on my chin. I look down to see Aidan has grasped hold of my finger with one hand and with the other he has reached up and brushed his miniature fingers against my chin.

Heart-warming joy is the only way to explain how I feel holding my son.

As I hold Aidan close, my heart aches to hold his brother too. I am afraid this will never happen.

***

The potent drugs Ethan is receiving have serious side effects—such as bleeding in the gut and calcium loss. A loss of calcium at this stage can interfere with bone development—even to the point of breaking bones and rickets.

Extensive use of antibiotics also brings a risk of profound deafness and damage to the kidneys. If the kidneys shut down, it is game over.

These side effects however, seem like a distant threat. The more urgent issue is Ethan's hypertension from the systemic blood infection. This is not responding to treatment.

The sepsis continues to spread and the massive dose of antibiotics needed is just a likely to kill Ethan, as it is to kill the bacteria.

The doctors are preparing us for a probable dire outcome.

My son teeters on the edge of disaster.

We are bracing for the inevitable news…so horrible I can't write the words in this journal.

***

Nana's dear friend Patty stops by for a lunchtime visit. My mother tells me—long after this nightmare is over—that this was a dark day for her.

Over lunch in the hospital cafeteria a simple question was asked; "How are the twins today?"

Nana found she couldn't reply. Instead a flood of emotion broke loose and she sobbed. Patty listened and was there for her.

Nana is a rock under stress, but even she can break.

I'm so glad she has a strong friend to lean on.

Our close friends and family have all stepped forward with kind words of support. Throughout this ordeal Justin and I have felt unrelenting despair—but we have never felt alone.

***

It's 9:00 PM. The doctors take us aside and say aloud the words that crack my soul in two.

They tell us Ethan is not expected to survive the night. His lungs are on the brink of full collapse and his blood gas reading confirms his systems are shutting down.

I don't know how I can handle this anymore.

I fear I am about to break into a million pieces.

While Nana places phone calls to family to let them know Ethan is in respiratory failure, I stare at my son taking in every little thing.

When you know time is running out, you try to fix things in your memory.

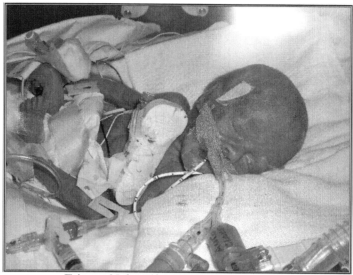

Ethan at 25 days old – 879 grams (~ 1 lb. 15 oz.)

Chapter 13 - *"Hail Mary"*

"Hope never abandons you. You abandon it."

George Weinberg

Friday, November 3, 2006
NICU Day 26

It's 3:00 in the morning and I have not moved from Ethan's side all night. The room is deathly quiet except for the steady swoosh sound of the ventilators and occasional beep of the monitors.

Ethan is receiving another blood transfusion and massive doses of antibiotics to get on top of the blood infection. His little body swells with fluid retention and his nose flattens out to just a little bump.

As Dr. Placket enters the room, I take a quick glance over my shoulder and see Justin and my parents have fallen sound asleep where they sit wedged together on the tiny bench like a row of disheveled rags dolls.

Dr. Lim joins us, and he and Dr. Placket talk softly so as not to wake my family. They say the antibiotics are not working. They fear that something is continuously re-infecting Ethan.

They counseled with infectious disease specialists and everyone agrees the source of the bacteria must be coming from one of Ethan's IVs. The mystery is, *which one?* Swabs of each IV site are taken repeatedly to try to identify which one is the primary source feeding this infection.

Our soft voices wake my family. Dr. Lim speaks up so everyone can hear his update. "The team was on the right path tackling the infection Ethan had two weeks ago; however, this time the infection is much stronger and it is taking too long to respond. This is considerably worse. I have serious concerns with the outcome.

He pauses briefly to check the IV flow rate. "We are fighting back with everything we have to knock this infection."

One look at Dr. Placket and Dr. Lim's strained but determined faces, and we know this is a tough fight they are not ready to concede.

Saturday, November 4, 2006
NICU Day 27

Ethan continues to teeter on the edge. His blood pressure fluctuates whenever he is touched; the DIC infection is not responding to antibiotics; and the doctors don't know which IV line is the primary source of the infection.

A daring plan is created. The doctors will remove *all the IVs* in order to save Ethan. It's daring because without an IV line, there is no way to administer medications or fluids. It's daring because once the lines are removed, there is no assurance they will be able to insert new ones. It's daring because if this fails, we lose Ethan.

***

At mid day the lab results indicate *yet another infection!* The tracheal culture shows a new Gram-negative bug is present. No more time to confer on the merits of the plan for IV swaps. We have to take action right now.

The plan reads like a script from the TV drama series <u>House</u> where actors each week solve a medical puzzle. Ethan's puzzle is to identify which IV is the main source of the bacteria—remove it—and then get a new line in without spreading the infection.

All of Ethan's IVs have to be removed. He has three different types: ART, peripheral, and PICC.

Ethan's ART line tested positive for bacteria; but is it the primary source? The ART line is hard to put in, so the doctors don't want to pull this one unless it has already failed. This line has been oozing blood for three or four days now, so perhaps it is beginning to fail anyway.

The ART line is important for taking instant blood pressure readings. Due to Ethan's life-threatening drops in pressure, he needs constant monitoring to immediately adjust the flow of medication.

Without this ART line, blood pressure can't be monitored instantly. They could take pressure readings with a cuff; however squeezing his arm every 30 minutes will be very disruptive. Merely *touching* Ethan sends his vitals out of whack; there is no way he'd tolerate a BP cuff.

And of course, a manual reading every 30 minutes does not provide the instantaneous stats needed to identify a precipitous drop in blood pressure.

The next part of the puzzle is Ethan's three peripheral IVs. These lines are inserted into a vein and are used to deliver meds. Some meds cannot be mixed together—such as antibiotics and insulin—so all three lines are needed.

Ethan's veins blow easily and the trouble is the nurses have run out of places to start new lines. If they pull out the suspect IVs, there is no assurance they can find undamaged sections of vein to insert three new ones.

Now the medical puzzle gets even more complicated. Ethan's PICC line may be infected too. The PICC is embedded deep into an artery in the core of the body, and the doctors haven't been able to tell if this is also infected.

The PICC is reserved for TPN nutrition and liquids. They can't feed Ethan or give him fluids without this line, and they can't put in a new PICC unless he is totally free from infection. It's a real Catch-22.

The doctors huddle in discussion as they try to figure out the best approach for eliminating the infected IVs and inserting new ones—and throughout this drama they have to keep a fragile baby from tipping over the edge.

***

A daring plan takes shape and the doctors reach an agreement. The plan is reviewed with sub-specialists from several hospitals and every contingency is crosschecked. The details are laid out and presented to us as the best chance for Ethan. Justin and I clearly understand the consequences if this strategy fails.

To me the plan sounds like a 'Hail Mary' football pass; throw the ball long and hope like hell it is caught for a touchdown. This is a desperate plan, but at the end of the discussion I agree. It has to work; otherwise game over.

The IV removal involves a series of steps that must proceed in a precise sequence, and each one depends on the absolute success of the preceding step.

First, the nurse will insert three new peripheral lines this evening. Assuming the nurse can find a spot for three additional lines, the next step is to pull out the old peripheral, ART and PICC lines.

Tomorrow antibiotics will be pushed through the new lines for a full day to try to get ahead of the infection. On Monday, a culture will be taken to be sure the new lines did not become infected. If the new peripheral lines are negative for bacteria, the doctors will insert new ART and PICC lines on Tuesday.

Ethan has to survive the next 48 hours with IV access limited to just three new peripheral lines. *They must not blow.* Any loss of a line will be disastrous.

Dr. Lesotho pulls me aside. He says he will support the team decision—but for the record, he is against it.

"I do not believe this is a best course of action. You should transfer this baby to Mercy Hospital. I tell you this. You must do this."

I stand here with my mouth dropped open in shock.

He stoops his tall frame, bends his head towards me and whispers conspiringly; "This is bold decision to maintain Ethan for the next two days with no PICC line. Ethan is too swollen from steroids. It may not be possible to find a vein. We cannot do this. You understand? Yes?"

I can't handle his whispered doubts. I *know* what is at stake. We cannot enter this battle tentatively. Everyone must be on board and believe this will be successful. Without this belief, we are doomed before we start.

The nurses tell Justin and me that we can go home—they will call us if anything changes. But there is no way we're leaving tonight.

We settle onto the tiny sofa in the NICU room and try to stay alert and keep an eye on Ethan. However, at some point we're both asleep sitting upright. Someone covers us with a blanket.

Sunday, November 5, 2006
NICU Day 28

I keep thinking of the strategy for the removal of Ethan's IVs over and over in my head. This has to work. If this plan fails, the chances of him surviving are next to none. The stress of the all-in strategy presses down on me. It's not fair to Aidan if Ethan doesn't survive. They're identical twins; they were meant to grow up together.

It's 2:00 AM and the NICU is quiet. The nurse has Ethan's isolette lid open to change the dressings on his arm as she readies him for the big IV switch-out that starts in just a couple of hours.

Slipping off the sofa bench carefully so as not to wake Justin, I quietly ask the nurse, "Is it okay for me to give Ethan a kiss?"

I've never kissed my son. I've never held him. The closest I have ever been to Ethan is my hand thrust through the holes in the side of the isolette.

She looks at me in absolute shock.

"You've never been able to kiss him?" she says incredulously.

The nurse doesn't say another word. She just brings me a stool to perch on and opens the isolette lid.

I lean my head in and twist my back so as to angle around the IVs and ventilator lines to get close to Ethan. Holding myself this way hurts my back, but I don't care. I don't ever want to leave his side.

Nuzzling Ethan's face and speaking softly in his ear, I give him the pep talk of a lifetime. He will face a big challenge in just a couple of hours and I want my son to know he can do this.

I would have stayed like this forever, but after 20 minutes, the nurse tells me she has to shut the isolette lid to keep Ethan's body temperature up.

At 4:30 AM Nurse Virika arrives. We have only a short minute or two to talk, and I want her to visualize a successful outcome. So I ask the first question that pops into my mind.

"Tell me the name of someone you admire."

Virika smiles and says this is an easy question. "It's my great-grandmother. I was named after her. She was a remarkable woman who lived in Norway where she helped mothers and babies escape the Holocaust."

"They tell me her name means *bravery*," she adds.

"This is good," I tell her. "Think of your great-grandmother's accomplishments. We need all the bravery we can find for this IV swap."

***

Virika is ready now to put the plan into play. There is no room for error. The pressure to successfully insert three lines into this fragile baby is on—and all eyes watch Virika.

Oh my gosh! She does it!

Ethan is a little pincushion. He has three old IV lines and three new ones. One of the new lines is just for his nutrition and the other two are for meds and for blood transfusions.

Virika was able to keep one arm completely clear as a future site for a new PICC line. For now, blood pressure readings will have to be done manually.

So much for Dr. Lesotho's worry the nurses could not get the IVs inserted!

***

We are five or six hours into the 'Hail Mary' plan to swap out the IVs, when Dr. Lesotho pulls me aside once again to say he has concerns.

What?

We've already pushed the launch button! We can't stop now. Why… why… why is he voicing doubts?

I refuse to participate further in this discussion.

Getting no agreement from me, Dr. Lesotho goes in search of my in-laws. Finding them in the Visitor's Lounge, he lobbies them to take control of this situation. He wants them to order the boys sent to another hospital for the balance of the IV swap and to undergo PDA surgery.

Does he doubt his own skill to handle this plan, or the skill of the rest of the team?

My in-laws corner Justin and me and press forward the argument to move the boys to another hospital. They strongly feel this move needs to take place right away or we will be responsible for our sons' death.

Stress puts words into their mouths that should not be spoken aloud. They are afraid and hurting, but I don't have the strength to hold them up. I can barely hold myself up.

I escape this verbal ambush and go off on my own to think. Finding my way to the main NICU desk, I engage the first doctor I see in conversation. Using all the casualness I can muster for my voice, I ask; "So what's your opinion? Should we move Ethan to Mercy for the remainder of the IV swap and schedule a PDA surgery?"

Her direct answer is blunt and comes without hesitation. "The IV plan is working. Besides, Ethan can't be transported. He is too fragile to be moved. If Ethan can't tolerate a simple transport—well, he certainly wouldn't survive surgery."

***

As the day progresses things are going better. By 5:30 PM Justin and I feel confident enough to run upstairs to the cafeteria to grab a sandwich. We manage this dinner break in literally eleven minutes—consuming our ready-made sandwiches in the elevator on our way back to the NICU.

Arriving at the boys' room, we see Dr. Lesotho's tall lanky frame leaning over Ethan's isolette. He is wearing a huge grin! Even his eyes are smiling. The doctor is so pleased the IV changes went well. It could have been disastrous; but so far, so good.

The new lines are in and the day ends on a positive note considering where we started from this morning. Justin and I are exhausted with the pressure of making life and death decisions. The strain has been unbearable. We've been up 72 hours straight with almost no sleep and very little food.

Seeing Ethan calmly sleeping, we head home at midnight for a shower and hopefully some sleep for ourselves.

Monday, November 6, 2006
NICU Day 29

Nana and I carpool this morning, arriving well before 5:00 AM. As soon as we walk onto the NICU floor, Dr. Lesotho confronts us privately.

"I consulted a cardiologist yesterday. This specialist agrees with me. It is imperative these babies be moved to Mercy Hospital for PDA surgery very soon. You must do this. This is urgent. You must do this now."

The outburst is startling. I don't know what to make of this directive. I thought the matter was closed. I don't want to this; besides, Ethan is too fragile to be touched much less moved.

Instead of directly challenging Dr. Lesotho, I take a coward's way out and say, "Let's talk about this at morning rounds with the rest of the team."

I know the other doctors will be present and I'll let them deal with his lobbying effort to move the boys.

***

My plan to make Dr. Lesotho explain his position for transferring the boys in front of the other doctors falls flat. He is kept busy elsewhere and doesn't show up at morning rounds.

The updates are underway in our room and Dr. Placket and Dr. Lim are telling me there is still a long way to go before Ethan is considered stable. There is no change in status and he is still a very sick baby.

More blood cultures are taken and we need to wait 24 hours for the results. In the meantime, Ethan is receiving another series of transfusions to flush out the blood infection.

Just as rounds are about to end, I make a meager attempt to resolve the communication disconnect I am having with Dr. Lesotho. But I am so tired and so emotionally on edge that I don't handle this very well.

I practiced ahead of time how I would broach this subject. I had an articulate and calm statement all ready to go inside my head. But instead, as soon as I open my mouth I awkwardly blurt out; "Are the boys to be transferred for surgery?"

As soon as the words leave my lips, I immediately sense the doctors' think that transferring the boys is *my goal*.

I have totally blotched it!

Before I can correct this impression, Dr. Lim quickly responds; "No. Ethan is far too fragile from infections to survive surgery. At best any discussion about surgery should wait until the lab cultures are negative."

"And it's at least another two days before lab work is available," adds Dr. Placket.

***

Nana and I find a private table in the corner of the cafeteria. Here we huddle to discuss this communication mess over a cup of hot tea.

How does a parent hear a consensus on the medical plan when there are strong differing opinions?

Does this lobbying to transfer the boys warrant attention or can we safely ignore this as a sideline drama?

Should we tell Dr. Placket?

In the end, Nana and I decide pushing for a change in communication style would probably not work. We chalk this up to cultural differences and keep silent. Besides, our priority is *results* … not warm comfy words.

Looking back, I now know I should have brought this to Dr. Placket's attention as the NICU Director.

Silence is a mistake I so very much regret.

Will my silence be a misstep that ends the life of one of my sons?

Chapter 14 - *Extraordinary Measures*

"The world is not interested in the storms you encountered,
but whether or not you brought in the ship."

Raul Armesto

The minute Nana and I walk onto the NICU floor this morning, Dr. Lesotho accosts us with his words. His once beautiful accent now grates on my nerves.

"I arranged for these babies to be sent to Mercy Hospital for PDA surgery," he says. "This is done. I have done this."

What just happened?

Did something sway the other doctors to agree with Dr. Lesotho?

Did he go to over their heads to force a transfer?

Wait a minute—I am supposed to be part of this decision!

I rush off to find Dr. Placket or Dr. Lim, but find that neither one is on rotation until much later today. Has Dr. Lesotho done this while Drs. Placket and Lim are off duty?

"Don't worry," says one of the nurses. "The transfer was pushed back a day or so to give Ethan time to stabilize. I think your transfer date will be in a couple of days—it's not today anyway."

I'm confused—and scared. To keep control of my worries, I go back to Dr. Lesotho and ask him if this was a consensus decision by all the doctors.

He bristles and responds with a short burst of technical points that evade my direct question.

"It is done. These babies will be transferred soon. Both will go in the same transport vehicle, and…"

I am on overload and feel faint. I have to force my mind to snap back to what Dr. Lesotho is saying.

"…the surgeon's name is Dr. Pulling. He will do the PDA surgery. The team at Mercy Hospital is very good."

He pauses for emphasis then enunciates each word very slowly; "I have made this decision. Your babies will be transferred."

I yell *Stop. Stop. Stop.* Then realize these words are locked inside my head, as I am unable to give them sound.

I want him to stop this—but I don't know what to say. What if my gut feeling is wrong? What if Dr. Lesotho has been right all along and surgery is needed? I don't understand the ground rules. I am usually a take-charge kind of person—but I am incapable of challenging decisions made by an attending physician.

What's wrong with me? Why am I indecisive? The life of my child is at stake and I feel so inadequate.

***

At midday rounds Dr. Lesotho notes Aidan's blood gas readings are good—so good in fact he is off the ventilator permanently. He'll leave Aidan on CPAP for a while, and eventually move his oxygen support down to the nasal cannula.

This doesn't make sense! Just a few hours ago Dr. Lesotho was insisting Aidan be sent to Mercy for surgery. Now he says my son is making dramatic improvement.

I turn to the doctor and challenge him.

"If Aidan can come off the vent for good—even with an open PDA—why does he need surgery?"

Dr. Lesotho sees my challenge as a mother's fear, and he gently responds.

"Surgery must be done now—before Aidan fails. This is the opportune window for PDA surgery before your baby fails again."

I haven't given up and I change my tactics.

"Is this really a sound move for Ethan too? He is literally just coming off the 'Hail Mary' plan of swapping out infected IVs. Why is there a rush to surgery for Ethan?"

Dr. Lesotho does not answer my question directly. He clasps his hands together and presses them to his lips as if to hold back from speaking his thoughts.

"This must be done," Dr. Lesotho says at last. "It has been arranged. I have decided."

Apparently the plan is in motion. The boys will be transported tomorrow and surgery is set for the next day.

I wonder; what was it that Lesotho said to the rest of the NICU doctors to successfully argue the case for transfer?

This must have been a tough call for the team to make. They can't do the PDA surgery too soon, and they can't wait too long. I trust this team and know they weighed all the issues before making this decision.

All the same, I have my doubts.

***

By late evening, Ethan blew every one of his new peripheral IV lines *at the same time*. This was one of the risks the doctors were afraid would happen.

Dr. Placket just arrived and he is working on Ethan to replace the failed IVs. Ethan's veins are so scarred the process takes two hours just to get in the first line.

Ethan is given a sedative to hold him still while the lines are inserted. When Dr. Placket is done replacing the IVs, he jokes saying, "I wouldn't mind a sedative myself after the past two hours!"

As he looks across the top of the isolette, Dr. Placket says with a soft laugh; "Boy, was Ethan pissed at being poked when I put those lines back in!"

I feel better with Dr. Placket calling the shots. He's the pilot whose experience and calm keeps the falling plane from smashing on to the ground.

Stress, *yes*. Panic, *no*.

Dr. Lesotho is handing out parachutes; but it is Dr. Placket and Dr. Lim who are landing the plane. I don't want to jump out—I don't want to leave Mission Valley.

Wednesday, November 8, 2006
NICU Day 31

Transfer to Mercy is underway. It is a whirlwind of activity and Dr. Lesotho is overseeing the preparations. He tells me that last night he moved Ethan to a ventilator, since the oscillator can't be used in a transport ambulance.

Blood gas readings are good, but Ethan's hematocrit is low—so another blood transfusion will be ordered when he arrives at Mercy. The lung scans shows evidence of chronic lung disease[20] in both lobes—and the right lobe is not fully inflated.

Dr. Lesotho switches to an update on Aidan. "The scan shows this PDA is slightly open. It could open further. Preemptive surgery is needed. You understand? Yes?"

This doctor pushed and pushed for the transfers. I wonder—what argument did he present to get these approved?

Lacking a miracle to turn back the clock on decisions made and actions taken—the transfers are underway.

***

---

[20] Chronic lung disease (CLD) represents the final common pathway of a whole series of lung disorders that start in the neonatal period. Generally, the first lung issues are bronchopulmonary dysplasia (BPD), a chronic condition that evolves after a premature birth; and respiratory distress syndrome (RDS), because of surfactant deficiency. Surfactant is the substance that keeps lung tissue from sticking together. Chronic lung disease is an extremely serious condition, which requires invasive forms of therapy that are not without risk. Mortality rates vary from 50% to 80% in the NICU environment. The aggressive treatment for neonatal lung disorders is often responsible for much of the chronic lung abnormalities that follow. Early lung disorders have consequences that extend into childhood and beyond. In addition, they are accompanied by conditions not limited to just the lungs—CLD is truly a multi-system disorder.

Mercy Hospital is an hour north from here. This regional hospital serves as the primary pediatric referral center for hospitals in a four-state area. They have a Cancer and Blood Disorders Program; a Craniofacial Center; Heart Center; Neurosurgery; Orthopedics; Pediatric Surgery; and a Transplant Center.

The hospital is massive. It spreads over 25 acres and has all the services of a self-contained city. They even have a school on the premises for children hospitalized long-term.

As Justin heads out to call on one of his client accounts, Nana drives me to Mercy. We are shown where to scrub in before entering the Neonatal Cardiac Intensive Care Unit. Here we meet two of the doctors, Dr. Burnstead and Dr. Mike—never could remember his last name.

This is a teaching hospital, so we'll deal with a different team structure than what we were used to at Mission Valley.

Dr. Mike is a Fellow, which means he is done with his residency[21] and is now specializing in neonatology. He checked on the boys when they arrived at the transport dock. He tells us, "Aidan handled the ride to Mercy just fine, but Ethan did not fare so well."

Being careful not to criticize, Dr. Mike's opinion is nonetheless very clear as he continues. "Ethan is not a candidate for surgery. He is too unstable and far too fragile for this procedure. What Ethan needs is medical care—not surgery. But since you're here, let's see what we can do."

Nana and I just stare at one another. We know too well what each other is thinking right now.

***

[21] Residency is a stage of graduate medical training. A resident physician is a person who has received a medical degree and practices medicine under the supervision of fully licensed physicians—usually in a hospital or clinic setting. A residency can be followed by a fellowship during which the physician is trained in a sub-specialty.

I can't believe how different Mercy is from Mission Valley. At Mission the doctors and nurses come to the baby's room for rounds and include the parents in care plan discussions. The physical layout places the baby at the center of everything.

It is different here at Mercy. The area dedicated to sick preemies is huge—as it combines the Neonatal Intensive Care Unit (NICU) and the Neonatal Cardiac Intensive Care Unit (NCICU) on the sprawling third floor. There are four or five nurse's stations placed at key intersections throughout this combined unit of 70 or so rooms. Parents are to find their way to one of these stations for rounds if they want to participate in status updates.

As a teaching hospital, the medical team is huge. Doctors, Fellows, and Residents-in-training all gather along with the nurses, respiratory therapists, pharmacists, and all the other specialists for rounds at one of the Nurses' Stations. There is no space for a team this large to gather in the baby's room.

It seems that everyone I come in contact with at Mercy is a sub-specialist focused on one part or another of the baby. Cardiologist for the heart, pulmonologist for the lungs, neurologist for the brain…it seems there is one specialist for every system.

The physical layout is definitely a medical-team centric structure; and I do suppose conducting rounds far away from the baby's room is necessary to manage all the specialists coming and going. However, I still prefer the updates to be done in the room with the baby.

The whole hospital is dedicated to sick kids. The sights entering the building are heartbreaking. Brightly colored cartoon characters adorn the walls of the main lobby, but what you notice first are the kids. Some have baldheads, some are hooked to IVs, some are confined to a special wheelchair, and far too many are just sitting with the blank stare of resignation as they wait—totally ignoring the storybooks, toys, and bright fish in the tanks.

Siblings seem to know the routine as they wander off by themselves to a designated play area; and the parents have a strained look about them that speaks of fatigue of sleepless nights and unrelenting stress.

We're here less than an hour and I already know the baby in the room next to ours is awaiting heart surgery, and two babies on the floor passed away just this morning. We're not supposed to know this, with privacy rules and all, but we can't help it. The news seems to ooze from the very walls.

The sadness of this place engulfs me.

***

As I sit in the lobby filling out admission paperwork, I overhear a parent on his cell phone. He looks young— maybe in his early 20's. This dad paces the floor in front of me as he talks into his cell phone.

I hear him say, "My son needs a stem cell transplant. My boss says I'm not eligible for insurance until I have worked for another six months. So I need you to sell my truck and my CD collection. That should raise about $15,000. See if you can't find someone to buy my snow blower and ..."

I try hard not to hear anymore.

I can't wait to get out of here.

***

We meet the cardiologist, Dr. Pulling. He will perform surgery tomorrow on both boys and takes this time to describe the procedure.

"Having a PDA is like fighting with one hand tied behind your back," he says. "This makes it hard for babies to fight prematurity issues. Most babies handle this procedure just fine. Recovery is fast...generally 24 to 48 hours."

Dr. Pulling flips through the boys' slim transfer paperwork. "I see multiple attempts of medication to close the PDA were used for both boys. I think these drugs should have been stopped after the second series failed. To continue to try this particular drug risks bleeding and kidney issues. When it fails, the simplest solution is surgery."

I am listening, but I am thinking these comments must be based on a typical preterm baby. Dr. Pulling has not even seen my boys. His counsel is solely based on reading a thin transfer file. Does he even know that Ethan did not handle the transport well?

Clearing my head, I tune back into Dr. Pulling's description of the surgery details. He calls this a ligation surgery—meaning the blood vessel is not cut; rather it is clamped closed. Each boy will be placed on their side and the surgeon will enter under the shoulder blade through two ribs, which are soft and not yet hard bones. The left lung is lifted gently aside so as to have a clear view of the aorta. A titanium clip is placed on the open PDA valve to crimp it closed. Titanium is highly resistant to infection, so it can be left safely in the body.

Mechanically, I go through my list of surgical risk questions.

"The risks are low," Dr. Pulling says. "They include bleeding, infection, and damage to the vocal cord nerve. That's because the location of the PDA is near the nerve endings for the vocal cords."

Dr. Pulling adds one more risk. "There is the potential to nick microscopic lymph vessels that can't be seen. These would leak body fluids into the lungs. Also, post surgery there might be need for increased pain meds; however most babies generally have less pain because so little muscle mass is cut."

I feel a sense of dread. This is a train wreck I cannot stop. This surgery is both my hope for my sons' recovery, and my fear.

***

Rounds are underway at the Nurses' Station. We have to wait inside our room until it is time for us to join the debriefing. When it is our turn, we expect one of the nurses will come get us.

Nana stands in the doorway watching for a nurse to beckon us to rounds. It's not too much longer when Nana sees a nurse giving us a frantic wave to join them.

Just as we get to the Nurses' Station, we hear a doctor say, "…and that is why Ethan is too unstable for surgery."

"We will let him rest and stabilize—no tests today. If Ethan cannot be stabilized for surgery, he'll be transported back to Mission Valley to wait until he is strong enough."

Dr. Mike speaks up next and repeats what he said to me earlier.

"I don't think Ethan can survive PDA surgery. He shouldn't have been sent here. This is a surgical hospital and what this baby needs is medical care."

This is just what Dr. Placket and Dr. Lim have advocated all along!

I feel this is one big mistake. I felt that way yesterday before leaving Mission Valley, and I feel this way today.

Thursday, November 9, 2006
NICU Day 32

R ounds are held with each shift change. We listen for our name to be called and then rush to join the debriefing. As our boys' discussion wraps up, Nana and I scurry away just as another NICU parent takes our place on the stools to hear their baby's update.

This process is awkward and it leads to parents standing in the doorway of their rooms waiting to hear when it is their turn. It is pretend-privacy, but no one seems to mind. We're all in the same boat. Our children are in this dreadful place and we are all desperate for a miracle.

When it is our turn at rounds, Nana and I take a seat on the two empty stools as the attending physician starts in with a long list of medical stats on our twins. We listen carefully, take notes, and have questions we plan to ask; but none of the doctors' pause long enough to see if I have any questions.

The many sub-specialists bustle in and out of rounds in such a hurry they leave the unspoken impression of '...don't interrupt me. I am too busy to linger here...'

This is beyond frustrating. I'm supposed to be the advocate for my children—yet I have no voice. Whenever I do speak up, I feel as if I am patronizingly dismissed. The doctor will give a slight pause, nod his or her head, and then continue without fully addressing my question.

There is an unspoken rule that parents learn quickly. It is a rule that expects you to *listen* at rounds—this is not the time for parent discussion. I know critical care medicine is not my training; but these are my sons and I need to hear *all* the details of their care plan.

How do I manage this? Do I force myself into the detailed discussions? I think not—this would be breaking from the norm and I surely don't want to be seen as a problem parent. I have everything to lose if the medical team feels they have to deal with a disruptive parent. So I try to fit in with this routine, and just listen and take notes.

As morning rounds continue, the attending physician adds her update.

"Upon check–in, Aidan weighed 1054 grams (~2 lb. 5 oz.). His heart scan shows a small-to-moderate PDA at 1.5 mm, with a left-to-right shunt. His other vitals look to be stable, and there is a slight heart murmur detected."

She scans the computer screen in front of her and adds, "Also, it looks like Aidan had six or seven apnea episodes this morning."

The physician looks over at me and translates her update saying; "The tests show Aidan's PDA is not open wide enough to warrant surgery."

Does this mean we can go back to Mission Valley? I hold this question back as the update quickly switches to Ethan's stats.

"Ethan weighed in at 885 grams (~1 lb. 15 oz.); down from his 910 grams yesterday. The dose of lasix to reduce fluid retention in his lungs has flushed away some body weight. His blood pressure is very low and it appears the significant hypotension may be because of the ongoing hydrocortisone drip. His oxygen saturation levels are low, so another blood transfusion (*his 18th*) has been ordered."

The doctor pauses in the midst of her update as she silently flips pages of Ethan's chart back and forth a couple times comparing entries. Her mouth drops open in surprise.

"I am blown away. This baby has had so many transfusions his blood type has changed from *A Negative* to the universal donor *O Positive*!"

She adds incredulously, "I have never heard of anything like this."

Of course the change is temporary. Ethan will eventually switch back to his own blood type of *A Negative*.

The doctor flashes a quick grin at me; then continues her update with the medical team.

"The lungs were tight and wet upon transfer to Mercy, and they have improved somewhat today. Ethan's ventilator tube is 3.0 mm—which is considered very large for this size baby—yet he still has a 50% leakage of air around the tubing. We don't want to insert a larger tube; as this just stretches the trachea even further."

"Ethan's echocardiogram showed a moderate-to-large PDA before he was transferred. Today however, the scan shows a small opening with left-to-right shunting."

She turns to me and explains. "This PDA is too small to warrant surgery; and regardless, his vitals are not stable enough to handle surgery even if PDA was an issue. He is definitely not a candidate for surgery."

The doctor ends the update saying, "I already spoke with Dr. Placket at Mission Valley. We agree there is to be no PDA surgery. He wants both boys returned as soon as they are stable."

***

Nana and I head back to the boys' room happy that surgery has been called off. A treat awaits us as we enter the room. Nurse Joyce has given the twins a gift of a bright blue Ty Beanie Baby™ stuffed bear. The boys are not much bigger than this eight-inch plush toy.

Nana also brought a present today. She made tiny knit hats. I am particularly surprised with this, as my 'mother-the-business-executive' has never knitted anything in her life! I am amazed she figured out how to make little hats. She tells me she used a small lemon as a model to get the size just right.

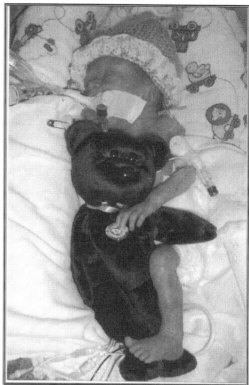

Ethan holding 8" Ty Beanie Baby Bear

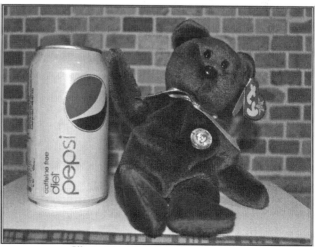

Illustrating size of 8" Beanie Baby Bear

The boys are awake and alert. Joyce has another surprise for me when she allows the boys to be in a single isolette for a short period. Joyce calls this *co-bedding*.

Aidan reaches out for his brother and clamps his little hand on Ethan's shoulder. What a sight to see both babies snuggling together.

I love it!

I think the boys enjoy this too. There is a bond between these two brothers we are allowed to see for the first time.

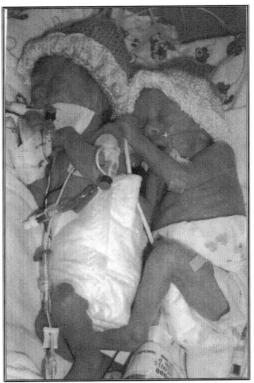

Ethan and Aidan – first time co-bed in isolette

Friday, November 10, 2006
NICU Day 33

We are on a rollercoaster ride. Yesterday the heart scans showed the PDA was small and surgery was cancelled. Now, the scans show the valve is wide open in both boys. I am told surgery is back on for Aidan; they will squeeze him into the first available time slot. Ethan, however, is too unstable for surgery.

Since no one is sure when a surgery time slot will open up, Aidan is left NPO (no food or water by mouth)—just waiting and waiting for an opening in the schedule.

I try to console my son holding him in my arms. Nothing seems to work. He fusses and cries non-stop for hours.

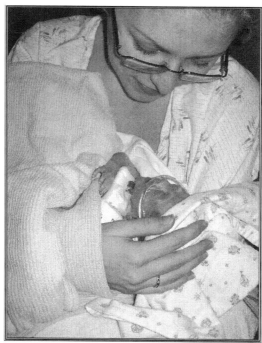

Mama holding Aidan before PDA surgery

While waiting for the schedule to open up for Aidan, one of the doctors stops by to provide details as to why Ethan will not be considered for this surgery.

The attending physician explains, "The standard procedure involves deflating the left lobe to gain access to the PDA. This is the only part of Ethan's lung that is actually functioning. Bottom-line, we don't think Ethan would survive surgery."

The doctor continues with an update of what comes next in Ethan's treatment plan.

"We'll focus on clearing the lungs of fluids with a steroid called dexamethasone—DEX for short. This steroid acts as an anti-inflammatory and immuno-suppressant. Its potency is about 40 times that of hydrocortisone."

"The nurses have a form for you to sign to give us permission to use DEX. And I need to warn you; if DEX is given over a period of more than a few days it can have many serious side effects."

He gathers his thoughts before continuing.

"Our goal is to stabilize Ethan so he can be safely transferred back to Mission Valley. I hope to have him stabilized by the time Aidan is recovered from surgery. This way both boys can return to Mission Valley at the same time."

This is a lot of information to digest while holding a baby that has been crying non-stop for hours.

***

You've got to be kidding me! It is way past noon and Aidan has been without food since the middle of last night. Have they forgotten they are dealing with a baby? They can't withhold feedings this long and expect to keep a baby calm.

What am I supposed to do? I can't find any one on the floor to tell me if Aidan is on the surgical schedule today or not. I have listened to my inconsolable baby cry since early this morning. I am about ready to start crying myself.

Finally, one of the nurses verifies that we will get the surgery slot that just opened up for 6:00 PM.

I wish I could tell my son this operation is to make him feel better and that I am so sorry for any suffering he endures. But all I can do is silently watch as they take him away.

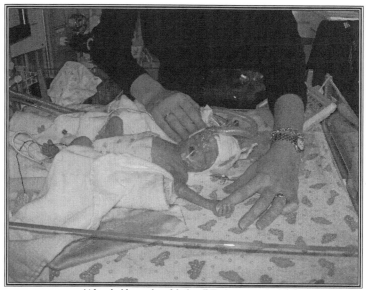

Aidan holds my hand before PDA surgery begins

Justin, Nana, and Papa are here. The four of us spend the next couple of hours sitting in the hospital cafeteria waiting for the pager to beep to let us know Aidan's surgery is over.

We stare at plates covered with half-eaten hamburgers. When the pager beeps, dinner is forgotten and we rush back to the Neonatal Cardiac Intensive Care Unit where the surgeon greets us with a wide smile.

"Surgery was successful. Your son is sleeping peacefully."

Saturday, November 11, 2006
NICU Day 34

Dr. Mike tries to listen to Ethan's heart. He asks the nurse to bring him a smaller stethoscope, but she tells him the one he has is the smallest size available.

"Great" he says with a laugh. "This guy is so tiny I can listen to the heart, lungs and bowels all at the same time!"

I like Dr. Mike. He is upbeat and brings a happy mood into our room each day. Even more important, he patiently describes the treatment plans so I understand how these will benefit my boys. And no matter how many questions I ask, he answers each with such detail I feel some degree of control in this horrible mess.

***

Aidan's surgery went well; however, he is still a bit groggy. He opens his eyes, recognizes me, and then drifts back to sleep.

Last night his chest tube had a healthy amount of fluid draining from the lungs, and this morning the drainage has tapered off. The doctors have Aidan on pain meds— morphine measured at 20 MICs last night and down to a measurement of just 10 MICs today.

They tell me they know how much pain Aidan has by monitoring his vitals. Right now his vitals are stable and he is sleeping, so we have to assume the pain level is under control.

By noon, Aidan's blood gas readings are great. He is already off the ventilator and back on CPAP. It's such a relief to have him off that damn ventilator.

***

There is also good news with Ethan. He continues on the steroid DEX to lower fluids from his lungs. It usually takes two or three doses of DEX before any improvement can be seen; yet Ethan's stats are responding positively after just one dose! The doctors were able to lower the ventilator setting from 65% all the way down to 30%.

The biggest news of all; *I can hold Ethan for the first time!*

I'm floating on air. Justin stops by—just as he does every day at lunchtime before returning to work. While I hold Ethan, Justin holds Aidan for the first time. What an amazing moment for the both of us. We feel like an actual family today.

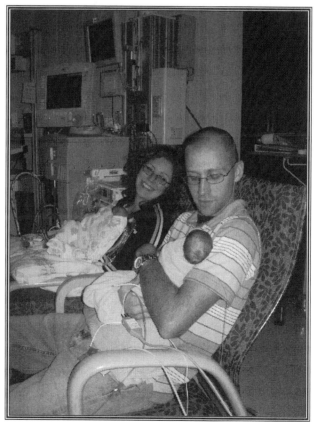

Family time!

Feeling so good after holding our babies, we head out of the hospital to celebrate with a nice lunch. We are not just husband and wife any more. We are Daddy and Mama.

***

The sixth floor at Mercy Hospital is set up for parents' use. The center of the floor has a large family area complete with several sofas, a big screen TV, reading material, and a row of four or five workstations with computers. I often see parents at these computers working their office jobs remotely—ignoring signs that ask users to limit time to 45 minutes per session.

There is a small kitchen with vending machines and a microwave. From the looks of the remnants in the trashcan, parents here survive on a diet of instant noodle soup and granola bars.

Surrounding the family area is a circle of hallways leading to about 36 sleeping rooms—each one not much bigger than a closet. This is where a parent can spend the night. Out-of-town families with siblings can try to get a room in the long-stay Ronald McDonald house across street.

Each sleeping room has a twin bed, a single lamp, and an alarm clock. Into this small space I cram my tiny overnight tote bag and the rented hospital-grade breast pump (it's so big and heavy it is fastened to a cart with wheels). There is no floor space left, so I have to climb over the end of the bed just to enter the room.

I crawl into bed exhausted and have barely fallen asleep when the fire alarm goes off. Staff direct sleepy parents to evacuate the floor, but I ignore them and go down the stairwell to the NCICU. I am not leaving my sons.

It is a false alarm. So back upstairs to the sleeping cubby and just as I fall asleep, the bedside alarm clock goes off. It is time for my 'every three hour' breast pumping session.

I reach for the lamp. *Click.* Nothing happens. The bulb is burned out and the room is so dark I can't see my hand in front of my face.

Grabbing a jacket, I plod back downstairs to find a light bulb; fix the lamp; finish breast pumping; and just as I lay down the alarm clock rings again. It's time to join the doctors for morning rounds.

Mercy Hospital's CEO stops by our room for a visit. He calls our tiny boys the "Miracle Micro-Preemies." We still tend to forget how famous these little guys are. Even in a hospital that treats the sickest of the sick, my tiny boys stand out as medical miracles.

***

Nothing much happened yesterday, so I skipped a day of posting journal entries. Today however, the doctor gives me mixed news. First, he describes Ethan's latest heart scan as showing a small PDA; noting blood is finally flowing in the right direction. The rest of the update however, is quite alarming.

The doctor jumps right in with the bad news; "Ethan's overall condition is unstable—too unstable to handle a transfer."

I wish Ethan had never left Mission Valley.

"Ethan's hematocrit reading is 21.6. This is down from the evening reading of 31.8. His red blood cells are dying off faster than his bone marrow can generate new cells. Another blood transfusion is ordered for today (*his 19th*). The IV in his head has blown; so before we can give the next transfusion, the techs need to find a viable spot to place a new IV."

"Chronic lung disease could be causing stress which opens the PDA. This is probably why there are so many fluctuations with Ethan's PDA opening and closing. The plan is to continue feedings and start weaning Ethan's vent settings. He had two very severe desats last night, and one again this morning which shows me Ethan still has a way to go to stabilize his breathing."

Despite the news that Ethan is too unstable for a transfer, I do hear good news in this update when the doctor notes; "Even with these desats, Ethan's oxygen is holding at 26%; down from the very high setting of 60% just two days ago."

***

Yesterday I tucked a small CD player into Aidan's isolette where it softly plays 'Baby Beethoven' music over and over. I figure this is better stimulus for a baby than listening to the swoosh sound of vents and the buzz of the alarms all day long.

I hear Nurse Joyce talking as I enter the room. She grins and says, "Aidan and I are discussing the merits of Baby Beethoven over Aerosmith."

She's a great nurse. When Joyce cares for my son, she treats him as a whole person.

I show her a game I made up with Aidan. I reach through the holes in the side of the isolette and lightly touch his lower lip with my finger. Aidan sticks out his tongue, smiles and looks intently back at me. I think he is studying my face through the plastic wall of the isolette.

Can he see me?

Does he know I am his mother?

I think so.

Chapter 15 - *Overdose*

"In the depth of winter
I finally learned there was in me
invincible summer."

Albert Camus

At morning rounds we hear the docs decide to change Ethan's sedatives. They will move him to a sedative and pain management cocktail of midazolam and fentanyl. The pharmacist attending rounds mentions this conversion is tricky; he'll need some time to research this.

I post these med changes to my journal—along with all the other medical updates—but I don't give much thought as to why they would want to change the pain med and sedative combination right now.

I wish I had. The change will prove to be nearly lethal.

***

Nana and I go in search of a quick cup of hot coffee and a muffin. The cafeteria food is not worth the energy to pick over, so we have become frequent visitors at the Starbucks located in the hospital lobby.

When we return to the neonatal cardiac unit, I can tell right away something is off. Ethan is unusually lethargic. He tries to open his eyes—they flutter open and close. Why can't he wake up?

Ethan isn't sleepy—he seems to be drugged!

Nana stays by Ethan's side as I run to find one of the nurses. The nurse however is not concerned—in fact she won't even come back to the room with me.

"If there was a problem," she says, "the monitor alarm would have sounded."

She blows me off as an unduly concerned parent and hurries off down the hall to take care of a baby in another room.

So here we sit staring at Ethan's monitors. Are we overreacting? Is there really nothing wrong here?

Suddenly, the monitor blares an urgent red alarm as Ethan's blood pressure plummets to zero and his heart stops.

Ethan is in cardiopulmonary arrest!

Nurses and doctors pour into the room and shoo us out. Someone grabs an Ambu bag from the crash-cart to manually force oxygen into Ethan's lungs to revive breathing.

We watch this frantic activity from the doorway. After a lifetime of holding our breath, one of the doctors comes over to us and says; "Ethan coded. I am concerned he might have been given too much sedative."

What's wrong with this elite team? I am glad they can openly discuss the error—but I am so mad. *An hour earlier* I told one of the nurses Ethan did not seem to be his normal self and I was dismissed.

I am pissed—I want to stand on a table and shout at them all. Instead, all I can do is nod my head as the doctor tries to explain what went so terribly wrong.

After several hours, Ethan's vitals stabilize. The crisis seems to be under control. I take a few minutes to talk with the doctors—but they have no answers that satisfy my question on the dosage error.

I want to know why Ethan was given the wrong conversion dose of narcotics. If the NCICU specializes in premature baby heart issues, wouldn't they have already figured out the formula for a proper dose of narcotics in a micro-size baby?

To fill in our understanding, Nana says she will research articles from the American Journal of Medicine. She wants to review studies on the use of sedatives and dosage conversions involving a neonate. Nana won't rest until she understands the physiology of what happened.

***

Nana and Papa return to the hospital at 10:00 to take me out for a late-night dinner. Justin joins us. He was dealing with clients all day and is anxious to hear the details of today's medical mix-up.

We takeover a corner booth at the local Olive Garden restaurant, and everyone is talking at once about today's mishap.

As we look over the menu, Nana debriefs us on what she learned on the difficulties of formulating meds for preemies. Apparently this has something to do with the extremely small size of the preemie and the ratio of body fluids-to-tissue mass, which is not the same ratio as adults or even full-term babies.

The hard part in coming up with a proper dosage is the drug manufacturer's studies show how drugs react in *normal body weight* patients. Calculating how an immature kidney and liver will process a drug in a micro-size patient is more of an art than an exact science.

The waiter brings us our pasta. Overhearing our conversation, he asks if we are doctors.

"No. We're just new parents," says Justin.

The waiter looks perplexed.

As new parents we should be discussing the merits of diaper rash ointments—not learning about drug absorption difficulties of fentanyl in a micro-preemie.

Wednesday, November 15, 2006
NICU Day 38

The boys have their first ROP[22] test to see if the vessels supplying blood to the retina are developing properly. Sometimes blood vessels in the eye do not grow correctly after a preterm birth and can cause blindness. This test will be repeated several times over the upcoming weeks and months until the eyes finish developing.

Although there is a correlation between preemies who receive high levels of oxygen and ROP, the doctor tells me there are other factors that may trigger abnormal blood vessel growth. These include small birth weight; early gestational age; elevated blood carbon dioxide levels; many blood transfusions; IVH brain hemorrhage; chronic lung disease; severe spells of apnea or bradycardia; and long term mechanical ventilation.

Well…both of my boys fit this high-risk profile!

As this eye test begins, the doctors excuse Nana and me from the room. We use this break to treat ourselves to a sugar-fix with a Danish roll and a cup of coffee. When we return, we hear the good news. Both boys passed the test!

***

One of the docs stops by and says Aidan has recovered sufficiently from surgery and can go back to Mission Valley

---

[22] Retinopathy of prematurity (ROP) is a potentially blinding eye disorder that primarily affects premature infants. The disorder occurs when abnormal blood vessels grow and spread throughout the retina tissue that lines the back of the eye. The abnormal blood vessels are fragile and can break; causing scarring and retinal detachment, which can lead to visual impairment or blindness. Infants with ROP are considered to be at higher risk for certain eye problems later in life, such as retinal detachment, nearsightedness, crossed eyes, lazy eyes, and glaucoma.

at any time. However, Ethan needs an additional 24 or 48 hours of DEX steroid treatment to stabilize enough so he can handle the transport. The doctor adds he is willing to keep Aidan here until Ethan is ready for the move.

We've been here longer than expected and I want to get back to Mission Valley. However, I absolutely don't want to separate the twins; so the plan is to keep both boys here and transfer them after a day or two.

I am still upset with the drug overdose episode. Seems to me the team relies too heavily on computer readouts and does not give enough attention to personal observation. If I told the nurses at Mission Valley '*Ethan looks unusually lethargic*', they would have believed me and taken action.

***

The day ends on a depressing note.

As I hold Ethan snug to my chest, I suddenly realize I am soaked with something warm and wet.

Has Ethan peed on me?

I look down and see a large circle of bloody fluid all over my blouse!

Ethan's arterial IV line is leaking and his blood and IV fluids have soaked through my layers of clothes—turning my white bra bright red.

No mother should have the experience of tossing out her clothes because they are stained with her baby's blood.

Thursday, November 16, 2006
NICU Day 39

When Nana and I arrive this morning we find the boys' room *empty!* No one warned us, so this is a momentary shock; but we quickly learn the boys were moved from the cardiac side of the floor (Neonatal Cardiac Intensive Care Unit) to the medical side (Neonatal Intensive Care Unit). Now that Aidan has recovered from his PDA surgery, the medical team will oversee the rest of our stay. We'll have the same doctors—but a new set of nurses.

The room we are assigned is an interior one. We'll miss the beautiful sunlight that filled our old room. Our new room is designed to hold just one baby and it is a tight squeeze to fit in *two* isolettes. The nurses have to jettison some of the chairs to make room. When there are two or more of us visiting at the same time, we take turns sitting on the single remaining chair.

Dr. Mike checks in on our boys and makes an endearing statement. "Typically preemies, especially micro-preemies, are really not very good looking. They normally look like shriveled aliens. Your son Aidan is actually beautiful; probably the most beautiful micro-preemie I've ever seen."

I am beaming.

***

Poor Ethan has been given nothing to eat all morning because *sometime* today they will get around to pulling his vent tube. It is not until one o'clock this afternoon when someone finally comes to extubate this little guy.

Ethan is hungry and crying so hard I am concerned he will now throw up any food given to him. And all of this crying puts so much strain on his lungs.

This is a phenomenal hospital, and I am in awe with what they deal with every day. Their processes however, place the medical team at the center of the schedule—not the baby. If the baby were at the center of the scheduling, Ethan would have been extubated first thing this morning so he could be fed right away. The medical team should have adjusted their work assignments so as to cater to the needs of the baby first.

***

I hate it here.

The family area sleeping quarters are not too bad during the day, but nighttime is terrible. Only the parents with the sickest kids get assigned a sleeping cubby to spend the night. The walls are paper-thin and all night long I hear gut-wrenching sobs coming from the other sleeping rooms.

Aidan is up to 1181 grams (~2 lb. 9.5 oz.). He successfully handled the nasal cannula all night and did not have to go back on CPAP. The doctors are able to stop some of Aidan's meds, as the frequencies of his blood oxygen fluctuation and irregular heart rate have slowed down. Recovery from surgery continues with no major issues.

Ethan on the other hand, has wide fluctuations from stable to unstable. He is very agitated and the doctors continue to give him extra doses of sedatives.

I'm not a big fan of sedating a baby—especially after the recent overdose episode—but it seems to be standard protocol so I stopped questioning this.

Ethan's CPAP pressure is at a mid level setting. If this does not work, they will try a high-flow nasal cannula before bumping the pressure up any higher. I sure do not like to see the settings creep up. I can just imagine this pressure adding to the damage in his little lungs.

***

There is now a third patient for my journal updates. I am sick with a fever and have an extremely painful lump in my breast.

My OB-GYN diagnoses this as mastitis and he calls in a prescription. I can't believe how painful this is and how sick I feel.

I dash downstairs to the hospital pharmacy to get the prescription filled—and when I return to the NICU, I immediately notice that the nurses have cranked up Ethan's CPAP settings one full notch. This extra oxygen pressure makes Ethan even more agitated.

What's up? I thought the plan was to use a high flow nasal cannula before resorting to bumping up CPAP pressure.

The mask of the CPAP has to be strapped snug across the face in order to create an airtight seal. Ethan hates this tight-fitting mask with a passion. I've been telling the nurses all along, my son does not like the mask and he will fight it. The more he struggles against the mask, the more agitated he gets and the harder his lungs have to work to breathe. As he fights against the mask, the nurses respond by cranking up the pressure settings. It's a vicious cycle.

***

I thought no one is listening to me. Surprise of all surprises…someone heard me after all. At noon the respiratory therapist brings in a high flow nasal cannula and it seems to me that Ethan finds this more comfortable.

Best news of all, the day ends on a fantastic emotional high. *I'm able to hold both boys at the same time!* It's the most magical thing I've experienced as a mother yet.

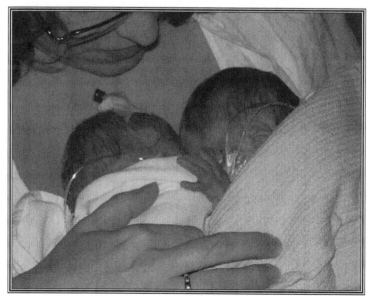

Ethan (left) and Aidan with his hand on his brother

Saturday, November 18, 2006
NICU Day 41

Aidan has his first bath today. A tiny plastic tub is set inside the room's sink and filled with an inch of warm water. I think he actually enjoyed the experience—alert and looking wide-eyed around his room. I wonder what he thinks of all this.

Bathing seems like an insignificant thing to post to my journal; but all mothers understand the importance of the ritual of giving their child a bath.

While the nurse helps me bathe Aidan, Nana is trying to keep Ethan calm so he won't cry. He's been fussy and hard to console all day. The monitors show his heart rate creeping up and up.

The nurse suggests co-bedding the twins to help calm Ethan's heart rate.

The co-bedding works! Ethan stops crying almost immediately when Aidan is placed beside him. The two brothers intertwine their arms, snuggle, and fall fast to sleep. I wonder; isn't this similar to the phenomena of calming a baby with the kangaroo-hold technique?

***

It will soon be Thanksgiving.

The annual drama of coordinating the holiday dinner with our parents won't be an issue this year. We plan to eat at the hospital cafeteria. I'll skip commentary on the hospital food as it will sound ungrateful—however, I just might smuggle in turkey sandwiches for our dinner entrée.

The nurse says with a laugh, "I have a nickname for your boys. I call them 'Bing' and 'Bong' because of the number of times they set off the monitor alarms."

The alarms sound in rhythm...bing-bong, bing-bong. As soon as one boy sets off an alarm (bing), the other one joins in (bong)! With two babies the alarms are pinging in stereo.

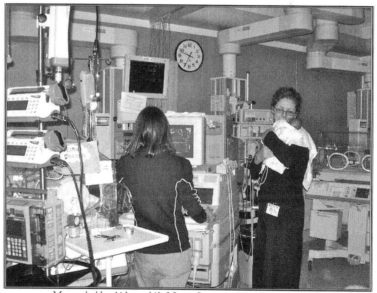

Mama holds Aidan while Nurse Jean monitors Ethan's stats

***

While the boys' genetics are essentially identical, I can see differences in their appearance. Ethan has been given powerful drugs to combat infections and CLD, so his environment is radically different from Aidan's. I can't help but wonder what other differences this will bring to the twins' mental and social development.

There are also mechanical differences in their care. The tight CPAP mask is strapped to Ethan's face for such long periods of time it is actually changing the shape of his head.

The respiratory therapist (RT) takes the oxygen mask off Ethan's face for a few minutes each day to give the eyes and nose a break from the mask's tight pressure. Otherwise it will rub raw spots. During these short breaks, the RT holds the tubing to blow oxygen gently across Ethan's face.

My son likes the freedom of no mask and he takes this opportunity to open his eyes and look around. I think he actually tries to *taste* the oxygen as he explores the air with a lick of his tongue.

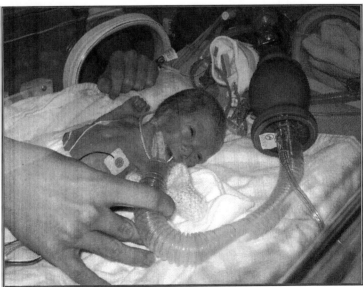

Ethan during a break from the CPAP mask

D r. Melroy gives us good news at morning rounds. Ethan is strong enough now to be transported back to Mission Valley. Five days ago the doctors thought Ethan needed just 24 to 48 hours to stabilize. It took nearly three times longer than expected, but we're ready at last. The transfer will be Wednesday or Friday. No transfer support on Thursday of course—that is Thanksgiving Day.

The doctor has more good news. Not only is Ethan finally strong enough for the transport ride, he doesn't think Ethan will need to come back for surgery.

"The PDA opening looks smaller and is not stretching the heart chambers. The blood is flowing in the right direction. I discussed this with the cardiologist and he agrees; this means no surgery is necessary."

I can't help but wonder. Would this have been the same outcome had we waited on Aidan? Did we rush him into surgery too soon?

While I am excited with the transfer plans, my ears perk up when I hear the doc say; "Ethan is on the pain medication fentanyl. Before we transfer him to Mission Valley, we want to move Ethan from fentanyl to IV drip morphine, then a final switch from IV to oral morphine. Drug conversion is complex in a baby Ethan's size, so I will research these conversions before proceeding."

This time I speak up!

"Why rush to switch meds if Ethan is going to be transferred to Mission Valley?"

My question is glossed over with a vague explanation citing differences in hospital standards related to these drugs. The discussion moves on to a myriad of other logistics related to the boys' transfer.

How I wish I could turn back the clock. I should have *insisted* they make no changes—especially changes right before a transfer that are described as very complex. It is too late now. Ethan will pay the near fatal price for the error that is about to happen once again.

***

By 6:00 PM I can tell something is wrong. Ethan is not himself. I run and grab one of the nurses. The monitors' show Ethan's stats are way off. He has a big drop in oxygen saturation down to 55% and his heart rate increases to 202—it should be in the range of 165-170.

The nurse comes quickly just as all of Ethan's monitor alarms blare in unison. She makes rapid adjustments to the vent settings and the stats seem to stabilize. She assures me everything is okay—probably just a little water in the line.

My in-laws have arrived with a surprise visit. They want to take Justin and me out for dinner. I really don't want to leave—I have a feeling I need to stay here tonight. Sensing my reluctance, my in-laws promise this will be a quick appetizer and then they'll get me right back to the hospital.

I am so tired I don't want to go; however the thought of eating something other than hospital food is appealing. Even so, I have an uneasy feeling about leaving my sons.

Instead of the promised quick appetizer, we end up at a fancy restaurant where they have booked reservations for a multi-course dinner. I know they are trying to give us a special night out, but I keep telling them; "All I want is a quick bite to eat so I can get back to the hospital."

I'm anxious to leave. I want to call the NICU to check on Ethan, but I am made to feel guilty that a phone call will spoil their dinner. I'm so preoccupied I can't hold up my end of the conversation and my in-laws surely thought I was rude. I am exhausted. I need to get some sleep.

The dinner finally ends, and Justin and I make the long drive home arriving well past midnight—far too late to get back to Mercy Hospital. I fall into bed but can't sleep as a wave of anxiety envelops me. I can't shake the ominous feeling that something is dreadfully wrong.

Chapter 16 - *Overdose Again!*

*"It's not stress that's the issue,
it's insufficient intermittent recovery."*

James E. Loehr

J ust as I do every morning, I swing by and pick up Nana for the drive to the hospital. This way we get the carpool lane and weave through rush hour traffic—shaving a few minutes off the commute. We head out early to time our arrival to be well before morning rounds start. First stop however is our local Starbucks. We're regulars and they have our coffee ready as we pull up to the drive-through window.

Arriving at the NICU, I sense something is dreadfully wrong. Ethan is intubated and he is back on that horrible ventilator. No nurses or doctors are near our room, so we wait for morning rounds to find out what happened.

Our names are called and we anxiously scurry off to join the team at the nurses' station.

The attending physician starts off with five words that send me into a tailspin.

"Ethan nearly died last night."

"The pain meds were switched from fentanyl to morphine," continues the doctor. "Ethan got his first dose of morphine last night and 40 minutes later had a severe apnea episode. His cardiac rate dropped down to 20, and then stopped. Doctors Burnstead, Searle, and Melroy manually bagged Ethan to get his heart rate, respirations, and blood oxygen back up. His condition remained critical from 10:00 PM to 1:00 AM…"

This was happening while I was stuck at that damn restaurant!

Did they over-sedate him again? If that's the case, how can they make an error like this? Twice! How can they have an infant in a major crisis and not call the parents? To hear all this at the morning rounds shakes my confidence in this team to my very core.

The update on Ethan continues, but I find it hard to concentrate on what is being said. My hands are shaking with fear and anger. Nana takes over the journal posting so I can reflect on the details later.

We hear the doctors say Ethan's blood sugars are elevated to 431. The norm is under 150. An insulin drip was started and this triggered a slow decline in his sugar level. Another blood transfusion (*his 20th*) was given to bring up the blood oxygen saturation. Ethan's heart rate remained unstable, so they gave him dopamine at 5:00 AM. His cardiac rate finally stabilized early this morning.

The doctors openly discuss this crash and say it might not have been related to the change in meds—rather it might be because of yet another infection. The high sugar level could be indicative of sepsis. Labs are ordered to confirm.

Other ideas are discussed. Could this latest crash be because of meningitis? A lumbar puncture is scheduled to rule this out.

In the meantime, until the doctors can rule out infection, *both boys* are placed in isolation and given a potent series of antibiotics.

Despite what is said at rounds, I am confident this crisis was because they overdosed Ethan.

We find out later my suspicion is right.

Damn it. This nearly killed Ethan.

This is our new reality—at any point critical care medicine is as apt to harm as it is to heal.

The transfer back to Mission Valley is called off again.

I am so angry it takes all my energy just to remain civil.

I want out of here.

Now!

Wednesday, November 22, 2006
NICU Day 45

Nana and I don't leave Ethan's room for rounds this morning. Our absence is noticed and Dr. Seaton, the NICU Chief of Medicine comes to talk with us. I ask her what triggered yesterday's crisis and she explains the possible causes.

"This could be due to an infection, or the switch from fentanyl to morphine, or the switch from a drip morphine to oral dose. We just don't know yet," she says. "We're considering all of these."

***

Nana and I stare at Ethan's monitors. The screens show FiO_2 is up to 50%, the PEEP reading is 24 to 26, and the pressure setting is holding steady at 6.0.

We're not sure what these numbers mean. When one of the residents comes by, Nana asks him to train her to read the vent monitors.

Taking up the role of teacher, Dr. Melroy says, "The FiO_2 measurement stands for Fraction of inspired Oxygen. The measurement is expressed as a number from zero (0%) to one (100%). The FiO_2 of normal room air is 0.21 (21%)."

He explains how the ventilator can be manipulated to mimic normal breathing patterns by changing not only the FiO_2, but also the tidal volume (the volume of inhale and exhale breaths); the respiratory rate (the number of breaths per minute); and controlling the amount of pressure present in the airways at the end of a breathing cycle, as measured by Positive End-Expiratory Pressure, or PEEP for short.

This is starting to sound like med school!

Dr. Mike has now joined the tutoring session. With the flare of a dynamic lecturer, he adds; "Before we can explain PEEP, we have to first talk about how the lung is constructed. The lung is made up of numerous branching airways. The tiniest of these airways are microscopic and end with small air sacs called alveoli. As the baby takes in a breath, the alveoli expand with air. This is where the exchange takes place as blood takes in oxygen and gets rid of the carbon dioxide."

Dr. Mike is animated as he continues his part of the teaching lesson. "The lungs are missing an important material in preemies. For the lungs to work properly, their lining has to be completely covered with a slick, soapy coating called surfactant."

"A growing fetus doesn't make enough surfactant to breathe outside of the womb until a certain point in development. Babies born prematurely have only about five percent of the total surfactant that they need; which puts them at high risk for respiratory problems."

Smacking his hands together, then slowing pealing them apart as if to illustrate he adds, "This surfactant is the stuff that keeps the alveoli from collapsing and sticking together between each breath."

Dr. Melroy cuts in again. "That's why we monitor PEEP. This is a measurement of the pressure used to prevent the lungs from collapsing. The pressure not only keeps air sacs open, it also helps recruit collapsed areas to re-open again."

All this seems like strange details to learn; yet this is just what Nana needs. Her way of managing stress is to learn everything she can—no detail is too small, no explanation too technical. She inhales this information as her way to gain control over an out-of-control situation.

***

Dr. Melroy returns a few hours later to perform the lumbar puncture to rule out meningitis. He got the needle into Ethan's spinal column on the first try and filled three vials with clear spinal fluid. Usually there is a slight tinge of blood in the fluid; however, if it comes out perfectly clear it is called a 'champagne pull'.

He laughs and says, "A 'champagne pull' means the Fellow has to buy the Resident a bottle of champagne!"

Looking just a little pleased with himself, he jokes, "Now I'm done torturing your boy, so I'm off to other rooms!"

Ethan never cried once during this procedure. After the lumbar puncture was over, a nurse comes in to change his diaper and he makes a big fuss.

Go figure!

Thanksgiving Day - Thursday, November 23, 2006
NICU Day 46

The results of yesterday's lab work are back. They show Ethan's throat is again coated with Gram-negative *Serratia*[23]. This bacterium can quickly become resistant to antibiotics, and if it enters the bloodstream, the bacterium will release endotoxins causing fever, septic shock, and DIC. We have been down this road before, and I am morbidly afraid of another bout of DIC.

I talk with Dr. Seaton to understand how this infection occurred.

"When we switched Ethan from fentanyl to morphine, the change in the medication was complicated," she says. "An error occurred and Ethan was overdosed causing his respirations and heart rate to fall to a dangerous level."

"To recover, we had to do an emergency procedure to get a ventilator tube down Ethan's throat as quickly as possible. This was a rushed procedure and when the tube insertion was done, it scrapped open a colony of *Serratia* lying dormant in the back of Ethan's throat. Since plastic tubing is the ideal breeding ground for this bug to grow, the infection spread rapidly to his lungs."

She waits a moment, as if to check that I am tracking with her explanation.

"Now that the lab results show which strain of *Serratia* we are battling, we can adjust from a broad spectrum antibiotic to a targeted set. If this works, we should see signs of improvement in two to four days."

The doctor is seated on a little wheeled stool next to Ethan's isolette. She stares down at her folded hands lying

---

[23] *Serratia* is a gram-negative, anaerobic (e.g., lives without oxygen) bacteria and it thrives in moist environments. Respiratory infections from *Serratia* are common in patients on ventilators.

on her lap. Looking up she adds, "Further spread is not likely, as this was caught in time and it should stay confined to the lungs as pneumonia."

The doctor pauses before adding; "This is a particularly troublesome bacterium, and we generally find it to be unpredictable. It could be a tough bug to battle. We will need to watch it closely."

I say nothing. I am afraid if I open my mouth a wounded animal sound will come out.

***

It has been a long day. Normally it would be just the nursing staff bustling in and out of the NICU room; but Dr. Seaton has not left Ethan's bedside all afternoon.

Nana and I are slumped together as we share the room's only chair. We have to wear the uncomfortably hot isolation gowns and masks. I don't think any of us has moved or said a word for hours.

Suddenly, Ethan's oxygen alarm pings sharply and Dr. Seaton looks over at us.

"It's okay—just inhale," she says to us as she reaches to reset the monitor alarm.

The doctor makes a few adjustments to Ethan's vent settings, and then resumes her position on the stool to continue the bedside vigil.

***

Today is Thanksgiving. My family—parents, brother and sister-in-law—join Justin and I at a small table in the hospital cafeteria for our holiday meal. Nana opens a large paper grocery sack and pulls out decorations she brought from home. She lays a placemat in the center of the table and fills it with décor. There's a tacky fake pumpkin, two unlit candles, and a miniature Horn of Plenty with plastic vegetables glued inside. It is as if she is trying to create a festive mood. This is so out of character for her. Nana never buys this kind of stuff. She must be desperate to create normalcy for our family.

The cafeteria food has been sitting in warming trays for so long it turns into a congealed mass on our plates. No one eats anything except for a slice of pumpkin pie that Nana smuggled in.

And we are thankful.

Saturday, November 25, 2006
NICU Day 48

Nothing was posted to the journal yesterday as I was so disappointed the transfer to Mission Valley did not occur. The logistics of scheduling the transport team around Thanksgiving did not line up.

We're stuck here through the holiday weekend. Nana and Nurse Jean (one of best-ever dayshift nurses), take this time to create a surprise for me. They make souvenir hand and foot prints of my boys.

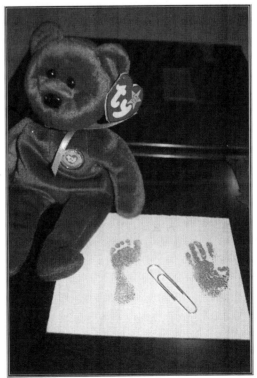

Aidan's tiny prints

***

The doctors at Mercy now understand that Nana and I need to hear the technical points of my boys' care—not just generalizations. So they adjust their communication style to be more forthcoming with details.

Off-line, one of the nurses tells me confidentially that the team is surprised at the amount of medical information our family seems to inhale—and understand. She says they're more accustomed to families wanting to leave technical discussions up to the doctors and nurses.

I want to tell her that NICU families' information needs vary throughout their hospital stay. But these words sounds patronizingly simple inside my head, so I just keep it to myself.

***

At rounds this morning, the doctors describe the implications of a baby left too long on oxygen therapy. A big concern is these babies can develop cerebral palsy.

To get Ethan off the vent, he is being given another round of the potent steroid DEX. The risk is high, and we sign yet another consent form acknowledging we were counseled on potential long-term issues of steroid use—such as hypertension that can lead to cardiac issues, decreased growth, and cerebral palsy.

We are told the vent can cause problems *and* DEX can cause problems. So what choice do we really have?

It's like saying you can choose the prize behind curtain Number 1 or curtain Number 2—yet the same bogey prize lurks behind both curtains.

Chapter 17- *Back "Home"*

"Hope is like the sun,
which as we journey toward it,
casts a shadow of our burden behind it."

Samuel Smiles

Monday, November 27, 2006
NICU Day 50

After 19 long days at Mercy, we are finally transferring back to Mission Valley. I'm so excited! The twins are safely tucked inside special transport isolettes and loaded into the ambulance. It's pretty crowed in there, as the boys are accompanied by a neonatal nurse and a respiratory therapist.

The driver is the nicest man. He flashes the lights and bleeps the sirens 'hello' as Justin and I follow the transport vehicle out of the parking lot.

As we begin the hour-long commute to Mission Valley, a quote from Charles Dickens pops into my head; *"One always begins to forgive a place as soon as it's left behind."* I respect the talents at Mercy and the wealth of possibilities their skill brings to sick babies. However, I am not forgiving of Ethan's two overdoses—not just yet anyway.

***

Arriving at the Mission Valley NICU, we are greeted by Nurse Julie and Dr. Placket. Julie gives me a big hug and Dr. Placket winks at me as he leans over Aidan's transport isolette.

"Wow, look at this big kid," he jokes.

Okay, I know Aidan is only three pounds, but it's all relative!

When the second transport isolette is brought into the NICU, Dr. Placket and several other doctors quickly begin their examination of Ethan. As I talk with Julie, I keep one ear tuned to hear snatches of the doctors' conversation.

Dr. Placket's tone is controlled fury. He wants to know what the hell happened. I overheard him say there has been no progress with lungs or weight gain while at Mercy, and Ethan has taken a step backwards from where he was 20 days ago.

What a treat we have this morning. I arrive to see Aidan dressed in baby clothes! It's the first time he has worn clothing. I am outwardly tickled with this—but I won't tell anyone I also feel a little twang of jealousy. I bought newborn matching outfits for my sons and dreamed of being the first one to dress them. I have to give up this experience to their other 'mothers'—the NICU nurses.

Just shy of two months old, Aidan is still too small for newborn clothes, so the nurse dressed him in a preemie size. The clothing hangs loose and I fuss with it by rolling up the sleeves and leggings.

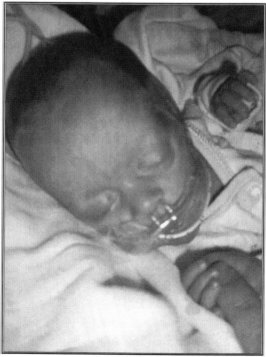

Aidan's first clothes

***

Ethan continues to struggle with his lung issues. Dr. Lim explains the situation. "Ethan's vent has another big leak. This is because the trachea has been stretched so much the tube is once again too small and air is escaping. If we step-up the tube size, it will further stretch his air passageway. We really don't want to do this. Changing tube size can become a spiral of ever-increasing diameters."

"Because there is an air leak, Ethan is actually receiving only moderate vent support. While the vent settings look like they are on a max level, so much air is leaking around the tube the actual amount of support Ethan is receiving is really at a lower range. This means he has lower oxygen needs than what the settings reflect."

This is a quality I so admire in Dr. Lim; he doesn't rattle off statistics without relating them specifically to Ethan.

As Dr. Lim continues his update, I feel the ever-present tension that grips my heart relax just a bit.

We are back 'home' at last.

The nurses post on the white board the boys' latest weight measurements. Aidan is up to 1470 grams (~3 lb. 4 oz.). The nutritionist will evaluate the feedings and weight gains and let us know if we can start Aidan on bottle feedings next week. It will be so nice to get rid of his darn feeding tube.

Ethan's weight is 1040 grams (~2 lb. 4 oz.). He had really good blood gas readings throughout the night, and his oxygen support level is currently at 30% (room air is 21%). If all goes well at this lower setting, the doctors can move him to CPAP soon. I monitor every change in oxygen support even more obsessively than I do weight measurements.

***

At morning rounds, the discussion picks up where it left off yesterday as to whether Ethan should have a larger vent tube. The backwash of air leaks continues, yet Dr. Lim is adamant about no changes in tube diameter.

"Do not increase the tube size," he says firmly to the medical team. "The one being used in Ethan is already considered too large for a baby this small. We need to be extremely cautious about any changes in this vent tube."

By 7:00 PM Ethan is no longer receiving sedatives—and he is definitively cranky! Nurse Julie is doing what she can to calm him with soothing words and a gentle touch.

She turns to me and says, "He's fine. Go on home and get some rest. Your boys will see you in the morning."

We head home; never realizing what is in store for us in just a few short hours.

Chapter 18 - *Respiratory Failure*

*"You'll be surprised to know how far you can go
from the point where you thought it was the end."*

Unknown

Thursday, November 30, 2006
NICU Day 53

C risis! Dr. Placket calls us at 2:00 AM. "You may want to come back to the hospital. Ethan is in respiratory failure."

I can't seem to catch my breath as I throw on some clothes. As Justin races us back to the hospital, I manage a quick phone call to Nana and Papa.

As soon as we arrive, Dr. Placket fills us in on the details of the situation. "Ethan is back on the oscillator. His saturations started dropping last night around 9:00 and Dr. Lesotho put in a larger vent tube. However, this larger tube did not keep the oxygen saturations from dropping, so Dr. Lesotho ordered another blood transfusion. Unfortunately, this did not help either."

"The x-rays show Ethan's lungs look worse than before he was transported to Mercy. Dr. Lesotho tried everything he could to keep the right lung inflated, but it collapsed anyway."

He pauses for several seconds searching for the words he needs.

"Ethan had several procedures done last night. He was moved from the ventilator to CPAP, and back to the ventilator. When he was put back on the vent for the second time, a larger diameter tube was inserted."

"Vitals fell rapidly and I was called in to assist. I had to take Ethan off the ventilator and I placed him on the oscillator to try to stabilize the lungs."

This news shocks me. Why did Dr. Lesotho put in a larger tube? This was clearly discussed at rounds yesterday. The docs all agreed; no increase in vent tube size. Could this larger tube have been the trigger to make him crash? Or was the larger tube necessary because Ethan's lungs had already collapsed?

My head feels like it is being pressed with a heavy weight. The pressure creates a vacuum that sucks up the words being spoken around me faster than I can comprehend them. I want to respond, but all I can do is nod politely with my mouth held open in disbelief.

***

Nana and Papa arrive shortly after us and Nana takes over journal posting throughout this unnerving update.

"I want you to understand the seriousness of this situation," Dr. Placket says. "Ethan's FiO$_2$ setting is at 1.0 (100%) on the oscillator. This setting is the highest it has ever been for Ethan, and it is the highest the machine can handle."

He is grim and repeats himself.

"At 100% the oscillator is the maximum ventilation possible—we have nowhere else to go."

Dr. Lesotho joins us now and says, "I believe this baby's crash is because of chronic lung disease."

Dr. Placket is less sure and offers his view. "It might be a mechanical problem that triggered it; or reflux from a feeding might have gone into his vent tube; or possibly this is because of rebound from the DEX steroids."

He continues with one more possibility. "Or it might be inserting a larger vent tube triggered yet another infection. We don't know yet what tipped Ethan's lungs to collapse again."

***

Things have not improved and by midday Dr. Placket is concerned with Ethan's lack of recovery. It has been over 10 hours and my son is still on the oscillator setting of 100%. Even with this highest setting, they can only get his oxygen level up to 70%.

This oxygen level is too little to sustain life for long. Dr. Placket makes a bold decision to move Ethan off the oscillator and step *down* to a regular ventilator. On the vent, Ethan's saturation level drops even further to 40%; then rebounds with modest improvement.

Ethan is given a small dose of DEX to pull fluid off his lungs. Dr. Placket is generally against the use of this particular steroid, but since Mercy Hospital used it for an extended period, he thinks the latest lung collapse might be due to the rebound effect of coming off potent steroids too quickly.

Dr. Placket was not scheduled for rotation last night— nor was he supposed to be here today. When Ethan crashed, he came in to take over my son's care. The nurses tell me Dr. Placket is supposed to be on an airplane right now headed to Washington, DC where he is scheduled to deliver a speech at a medical conference *against* the prolonged use of DEX.

I ask Dr. Placket about this conference, but he just shrugs as if this national meeting is not important.

"I'll catch another flight—or maybe not. I am not leaving Ethan right now."

***

The lung crisis continues in the evening hours. The NICU room is packed with nearly the entire medical team hovering over Ethan. Everyone is quiet as they study vitals and monitor the machines.

Justin and I sit silently on the little sofa bench, while Nana and Papa perch on either end as if they are protective bookends holding us safely upright.

We are paralyzed with fear. Has Ethan come this far only to lose his battle now?

Just before midnight we head home, as there is no place for us to sleep at the hospital tonight.

We should have stayed. The next crisis will arise in less than three short hours.

It is midnight when we finally get home and fall into bed exhausted. We're not asleep long before the phone rings. It's 2:30 AM—and Dr. Lim is saying Ethan has crashed again. The right lung collapsed for the second time in the past 24 hours. I go into a full panic attack. I cry and shake and try not to hyperventilate as Justin drives us back to the hospital.

Dr. Lim meets us at Ethan's bedside. He says it was a good thing they had already put in the ART and extra peripheral lines yesterday. Ethan's veins are so collapsed he's not sure they could have gotten any new IVs started today.

Ethan received two urgent blood transfusions (*his 22nd and 23rd*) in the wee AM hours. The blood gas is showing improvement, so they weaned back the FiO_2 to 54%. That's a good number compared to the 100% support needed last night.

***

Nana and Papa arrive just a few minutes after us, and Dr. Lim pulls all of us aside for another update.

He gently explains, "There is extensive collapse of the right lung and Ethan continues to be very unstable."

"Yesterday, the oscillator was used to recruit the right lung, but in doing so it over-inflated the left lung. It was a brilliant move on Dr. Placket's part to take Ethan off the oscillator. The right lung was not responding and the machine was damaging the left lung—and the left lobe is the only lung tissue Ethan has which is actually working. It was both a gutsy and genius move to pull Ethan off that oscillator."

His voice sounds tight as if he is trying to control his tone when he adds, "The new tube Dr. Lesotho had to insert is considered very large for this size baby. I am concerned this tube is hyper-extending Ethan's trachea. This presents a troubling situation and I believe..."

Dr. Lim abruptly stops mid-sentence and changes direction with the update as he moves on to what will happen next.

"I expect Ethan could be on the vent for another week before he is ready to step down to CPAP. For now, nutrition is needed to help re-grow new lung tissue—and I have Ethan on a high calorie formula packed with carbohydrates, fats, and protein."

"There is a direct correlation between body length and new lung tissue growth," he says. "The more we can get Ethan to grow in body length, the more new lung tissue he will generate."

Dr. Lim looks grim as he ends the update saying, "Overall Ethan is a very fragile baby and we are a long way from being out of the woods."

Nurse Joan joins the NICU dayshift to fill in after Modra rotates to new assignment with the Pediatric Outpatient Clinic. Now nurses Julie and Joan are part of the team who take care of my boys during the day. These phenomenal nurses are my lifelines. I quickly form a bond of trust with them.

Joan is a tall athletic looking woman in her late 30's, and has many years of NICU experience. She has a wonderful way with words that leaves me feeling both informed and empowered in the care of my babies.

At morning rounds she starts off the update telling me, "This little guy has lots of goobers. I have to suction him frequently to keep the lungs open. Don't worry—this is a good sign as secretions mean the lungs are draining. The cells in the lungs are doing their job to move the gunk up and out."

The doctor on rotation today continues the update with the best news of the morning. "Ethan's x-ray shows both lungs are inflated and not hyper-extended!"

Adding more good news, the doctor says, "Ethan's stats are getting better. His blood gas shows the CO_2 level dropped down to 49—which is getting closer to the target range of 35 to 40. His oxygen support is 37%, the PEEP was turned down from 7.0 to 6.0, and the rate was turned down from 55 to 45. These are all good numbers. The game plan today is no major changes—just let Ethan dictate his own pace."

As I breathe in deeply savoring this good news, I look around the room. Something is different.

It dawns on me! The NICU room is decorated with Christmas stockings, and each baby has a tiny brown teddy bear sitting on top of their isolette wearing a gift tag; "From Santa." I forgot. It will soon be Christmas.

Sunday, December 3, 2006
NICU Day 56

Drum-roll please—Aidan's nasal cannula is removed this morning and he is breathing room air! For the first time in his life, Aidan is breathing unassisted. A baby book milestone; *on his 56ᵗʰ day of life my son breathes on his own.*

There is one more milestone for the baby book; Aidan has his first bottle-feeding. The bottle and nipple are so tiny they look like a toy. After this feeding his oxygen saturation level dropped, as it's hard for him synchronize eating and breathing at the same time.

Another drum-roll—this one is for Ethan. The x-ray finally shows both lobes of his lungs are at least partially inflated. They might not be 100% open, but partial is better than collapsed. What a strange thing to celebrate.

Ethan is getting his morning therapy session to move secretions out of his lungs. This therapy is a series of massage percussions and vibrations against his back to help loosen the gunk that fill his lungs. The therapist uses a suction tube to pull out the loose secretions. Ethan likes the massage, but he sure hates the suctioning.

***

Before we leave this evening, Dr. Baillie stops by. "If we can't get Ethan off the vent soon," he says, "this baby may face more severe issues. We may need to consider a tracheostomy."

He tells me trach surgery involves inserting a breathing tube into the base of Ethan's throat and connecting it to an oxygen tank. The typical trach treatment lasts for a year or longer.

I know he is helping us to manage our expectations—but when will this all end?

Monday, December 4, 2006
NICU Day 57

Medicaid finally got back to me today. It has been nearly two full months waiting to hear from them. I learn we qualify for an unspecified amount of help because the boys are considered disabled due to their extremely low birth weight.

Medicaid will supplement our insurance coverage as long as the boys remain hospitalized. It's not clear *how much* help they will provide; however they do make it abundantly clear—once each boy is discharged from the hospital, we will not be eligible for any more assistance.

The twins aren't even two months old and the bills are already over one million dollars. I am under the *mistaken* impression the hospital bills will be covered in full between my comprehensive health insurance policy and Medicaid. It is good that I believe this, because if I knew the truth I'd be seriously depressed.

It will be much later, long after the bills have piled up, that I will learn of exclusions in my employer's medical insurance plan and of the coverage gaps in Medicaid. These exclusions and gaps will leave crushing balances of unpaid medical bills that total more than *four times* our annual salary.

Today however, I have a more urgent problem to deal with. As I write checks for our household bills, I am shocked to see we are rapidly running out of funds to pay routine expenses. Two months ago our savings account had enough of a cushion to cover a full year of living expenses—but this is nearly all gone. I had to use a large portion of our savings to pay medical bills.

How will we keep afloat?

Chapter 19 - *Eat and Breathe*

"Family faces are magic mirrors.
Looking at people who belong to us,
we see the past, present, and future."

Gail Lumet Buckley

Tuesday, December 5, 2006
NICU Day 58

Aidan is bottle feeding several times a day. He can latch on and is learning to suck, swallow, and breathe without choking. I have to frequently remove the nipple when his mouth fills with milk, as he sometimes forgets to swallow and breathe at the same time.

Some new moms brag their two-month-old baby can turn over. I can brag my two-month-old baby is learning to swallow and breathe at the same time.

Aidan is still too small to regulate his own body temperature, so he needs to stay in the isolette for now. As he gains weight he will be able to handle room temperatures and move to an open crib—a big step before he can be considered ready for discharge.

Nurse Joan leans around the bulky isolette to peek at me and says with a big grin, "Aidan weighed in at 1646 grams (~3 lb. 10 oz.)! I weighed him *three times* because I just couldn't believe he weighs this much."

***

At morning rounds the stats for Aidan are all good. Dr. Placket flashes a big grin and says, "If Aidan's remarkable progress continues on this path, he could be discharged in three to four weeks."

My baby can come home!

What a strange thought. Instead of thrilling me, a pang of fear flutters in my gut. How can I take care of a three-pound baby by myself? He has needed all these doctors and nurses and therapists for so long. How can I do this by myself?

Of course, the updates on Ethan don't have any mention of possible discharge.

The doctors tell me Ethan's x-ray shows the lung on the right side is not open as much as it was yesterday and both sides are cloudy again with fluid.

They review again with me the possibility of needing a trach. I get the sense that a textbook approach for a baby with Ethan's symptoms would warrant a trach. It seems to be just the thinnest thread of hope that keeps the doctors in favor of holding off on the trach decision a little bit longer.

The docs are clear with their firm warnings. Ethan can't continue with DEX steroids for much longer, and he certainly can't stay on ventilators forever. If my son can't be moved off the vent soon, the next step will be a tracheostomy.

***

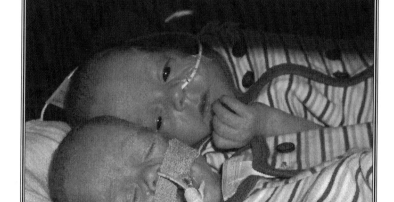

2006 Christmas photo – Aidan awake and Ethan sleeping

I take a break from all this stress and plan the first annual Christmas photograph of my sons. I want to dress them in matching outfits, but Ethan can't wear clothes because of his numerous tubes and IVs. So I just drape the preemie size outfit across the top of him and consider that good enough.

Nurse Modra stops by on her day off to say hello. I recruit her to help me with the photo session.

She holds Aidan suspended inside the isolette next to Ethan (who manages to sleep through the entire affair).

While Modra holds Aidan, I aim the camera lens through the armhole in the side of the isolette and squeeze off a rapid series of pictures with the flash turned off.

Sure hope this works.

What a mother won't do to get a picture of her sons for the family Christmas card!

Not your typical holiday photo, but I thought my boys looked beautiful.

Wednesday, December 6, 2006
NICU Day 59

Dr. Baillie evaluates Aidan this morning. He looks closely at reflexes, muscle tone, and movement. So far there are no concrete signs of cerebral palsy. Autism and other social or learning issues won't show up until later, so the plan is to test for these at another time.

Aidan, at two months of age, is steadily gaining weight. He's up to a whooping 1704 grams (~3 lb. 12 oz.). Close now to a full four pounds.

Ethan is usually very fussy in the mornings and today is no exception. Dr. Baillie finally gives up trying to complete his exam and says he'll come back in the afternoon. I can relate. I'd be cranky too if first thing in the morning someone poked me!

After the doctor leaves, I help Aidan relax by giving him a warm bath. I take special notice of the scars on his feet, arms, and wrists. These are thick white lines of scar tissue from the many IVs and an angry red scar across his back from the PDA surgery. I call them 'dragon bites.' They are battle scars Aidan earned taming the NICU dragons.

***

Dr. Baillie returns this afternoon to finish his exam of Ethan. This little guy has gained some weight. He is up to 1160 grams (~2 lb. 9 oz.). Just imagine—a two-month-old baby weighing two pounds. He looks much heavier however, as he is swollen with fluid retention caused by the continued heavy doses of steroids.

"Ethan's ultrasound shows a resolving brain bleed, which is noticeably smaller in size. And there are some cysts around the clot, which may be indicative of cerebral palsy," Dr. Baillie says as he takes a seat on the stool next to me.

"The small cystic areas are called PVL, and this is a normal progression for resolving clots. Some of Ethan's muscle movements are not well controlled, so I am watching this closely. It might be a sign of cerebral palsy, or it might be nothing at all."

The doctor gives my hand a reassuring squeeze, but all I hear are the words "...*cerebral palsy.*"

The words hang heavy on my heart.

Both boys have another eye exam today. The test shows their eyes are still immature and so far have no signs of ROP. Since the eyes are still forming, another exam is set for a week out. This is just a routine repetitive test. I give it nothing more than a passing note in my journal. I should have been more concerned. We'll find out soon enough another disaster is lurking and will land squarely on Ethan.

***

I sit slumped on a chair next to Ethan's isolette and stare at the monitor. The oxygen stats look good. In fact, so good the support settings are low and vitals are stable. I'm so preoccupied staring at the mind-dulling numbers flash across the screen that I don't hear Dr. Baillie and Dr. Lesotho come into the room.

Both doctors stand still until I am aware of their presence.

Pointing at the monitors Dr. Baillie comments, "Look at those great numbers! Ethan's stats are stable enough that we're considering extubation to CPAP as early as tomorrow."

This good news barely leaves his mouth when a red alarm beckons urgently from a room across the hall and Dr. Baillie hurries away to attend to another baby.

My millisecond celebration of this good news ends as Dr. Lesotho continues the update solo.

He's not focused on the lungs; rather he wants to talk about yesterday's brain scan. His words fill the room with blunt statistics and suck the celebration from my heart.

"Finding PVL cystic granules is bad news. These cysts are in an area of the brain controlling movement. I believe

Ethan may have cerebral palsy. I have placed orders for MRI to measure if this is so. You understand? Yes?"

This is similar to what I heard yesterday, but Dr. Lesotho's heavily accented words are more ominous. His concerns sound more like an affirmed diagnosis.

I hope it's just my strained emotions erroneously filtering how I hear the news.

My brain is not able to process complex sentences.

Every word seems to be muddled.

I am so very tired.

Tell me *now* how this journey will end and let me get on with my life.

Friday, December 8, 2006
NICU Day 61

Having heard Dr. Lesotho's view yesterday on the PVL cysts, I ask Dr. Lim today for his opinion. His words are sobering.

"The scan shows injury to some of the brain tissue; it's an area with cysts. The problem is, cysts don't fit with a Grade II hemorrhage—they are more commonly associated with a Grade III. The cysts are periventricular leukomalacia, or PVL for short. This puts Ethan's possibility for developing movement disorders at a much higher risk."

He knows Nana likes to hear the details on medical issues so he adds, "The term periventricular refers to the location in the ventricles of the brain and leukomalacia means an abnormality of white brain tissue."

"We don't know what the presence of the cysts will mean specifically for Ethan. All we know is statistically some children with similar issues develop cerebral palsy, and some do not. The developing brain is an amazing organ. It can compensate in ways we can't imagine or predict—we'll just have to wait and see."

I know this is of some concern for Justin. His dreams of teaching his sons Aikido, snowboarding, and soccer may be dramatically altered.

The uncertainty of this is so unsettling. I have to push it out of my mind for now. We can't do anything about it anyway.

Like everything else we've encountered on this NICU journey, we'll find a way to handle whatever we are dealt.

Just let me get my sons home.

Please.

Saturday, December 9, 2006
NICU Day 62

It's a quiet day today. No crisis, but no progress either. I feel locked in place with no end in sight—just sameness.

A wave of emotion is pulling me under.

I can't write.

I can't think.

I can't breathe.

The tears start to flow.

Monday, December 11, 2006
NICU Day 64

Two days ago I lost it. I let my guard down and all my pent up emotions pushed me over the edge. Funny thing about this—it was a quiet afternoon and the boys were stable. There was no crisis. There was no tipping point.

I grieve for the first time. I grieve for the loss of my pregnancy. I grieve for my chance to deliver my babies and experience holding them in my arms on the day they were born. I grieve for the life we dreamed of as we planned our family.

Where is the boundless joy that comes with being a new mother?

I miss my life. I miss who I was. I am afraid of what I am becoming. I feel like I am jumping from one tiny iceberg to another. Each one is smaller than the last. And the one I stand on now is so small it barely holds me up. I don't see any more ice chunks to jump to. If I fall into the freezing ocean waters, it will be an instant game over. I will lose my sons.

My OB-GYN says I am experiencing post-partum depression and traumatic stress anxiety.

I never thought I would be the one to crumble.

Tuesday, December 12, 2006
NICU Day 65

A rumor is floating around the NICU—Aidan is doing so well he may be able to come home in a few weeks! It is exciting to think we'll finally have one baby home—perhaps even by Christmas. Part of me can't wait to get him home, and part of me doesn't want him to leave Ethan behind. I worry about Ethan not doing as well without his brother by his side. After all, they are 'Bing' and 'Bong'!

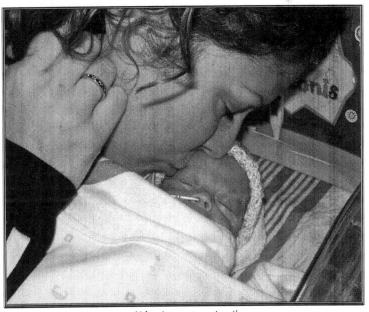

Aidan in an open-air crib

Several days ago orders were written to wean Aidan to an open-air crib. To prepare for this, the heat in his isolette was moved closer and closer to room temperature. By late today our big boy graduates to a crib. It's not your typical baby crib—it is just a small open plastic box.

It is so good to be able to kiss him whenever I want.

Thursday, December 14, 2006
NICU Day 67

E than is getting two more blood transfusions (*his 24th and 25th*) as they try to keep up his blood oxygen level up in preparation for moving him from the ventilator to CPAP. He looks good after the transfusions—they pink up his pale skin.

By early afternoon, Dr. Lim is back to deliver the latest brain scan results. "Ethan's brain cysts are static, meaning the cysts present now are permanent. Ethan won't have any more cysts develop; however the ones he has now won't go away. Damage done by these cysts is not a major concern because the baby's developing brain can make phenomenal progress to adapt and develop alternate paths."

He elaborates; "Contrast this with an adult where the brain has stopped growing. In an adult, cysts like these would cause permanent damage to motor, speech, or cognitive skills."

Dr. Lim balances these updates with empathy. I understand what he is telling me. I know he is not making absolute promises, but his words leave the door open just enough that I see the slim light of hope.

When Ethan reaches his arms up towards me, I believe his movements are intentional. However, there are times when I have my quiet doubts. Too often I have seen my son's head flop to one side and his arms and legs jerk with uncontrolled movements.

Chapter 20 - *Lights Out*

"When you have exhausted all possibilities,
remember you haven't"

Thomas Edison

Friday, December 15, 2006
NICU Day 68

Massive windstorms knock power out all over the region. Over a million customers are without electricity, and many roads are blocked with downed trees and power lines. The normal 45-minute drive to the hospital took Justin and me over three hours. Most of the hospital staff stayed overnight, knowing they would not be able to navigate the roads to get home. They also stayed knowing others would not be able to get in to work this morning.

Of course the hospital has backup generators—but the patient rooms and hallways are dark. It's eerie. We use a flashlight as we wander the hall to the restroom. The cafeteria is closed and the vending machines were emptied of food a long time ago.

What I wouldn't give for a cup of *hot* coffee.

In the dim light of the auxiliary power, I can see Dr. Lesotho's long angular face is flush with a big toothy grin.

He says the words I so longed to hear.

"Aidan looks great. Your baby can go home next week!"

It is a thrill to think we can have him home before Christmas. This news comes with mixed emotions. I've said this many times; I don't want to leave Ethan behind. And I am certainly not taking Aidan home until the power is back on!

Saturday, December 16, 2006
NICU Day 69

Power outages continue across the region and the hospital is still on backup generators. News reports say it may be another five days before the city has full power restored. The outlying areas may have to wait 10 days or longer. We live in one of those outlying neighborhoods and I am frantic. There is no power at our house and my freezer holds a two-month supply of precious breast milk.

No power also means no heat, no hot showers, and no hot food. It's hard to find a gas station still operating. When one does find a rare gas station open, there will be a line of cars spilled down the street as drivers wait to buy a few gallons of scarce gasoline.

Justin went out to find ice for our freezer. Hours later he is back. He had no luck; now our car has only a quarter of a tank of gas left. I think we're going to lose the entire supply of breast milk. It is so sad to have worked around the clock to pump milk and lose it to a power outage. This was the one thing I could do for my sons—and we're going to lose it all.

More hospital staff made it in today, but it is still a very lean crew. Several stayed over for the second night, as many have no way to get home. Everyone looks a little scruffy around the edges living in the same clothes now for nearly 72 hours.

As a long-timer at the hospital, I am informally recruited to help the short-handed nursing staff with routine chores. It feels good to be useful.

Now where the heck is a flashlight!

Sunday, December 17, 2006
NICU Day 70

Looks like a disaster movie-set with debris and downed power lines everywhere. While the power has finally been restored at the hospital, the rest of the city—and suburbs—are still dark.

Our bedroom skylight blew off during the windstorm and the rains drenched everything in sight. What a mess. We have towels laid out everywhere trying to soak up the water. Jameson the dog thought he was to blame for the wet carpets and hid until he realized he was not in trouble.

***

Another update of bad news is delivered at morning rounds. We hear one of Ethan's IV sites blew during the night and the doctor couldn't get another line started. She tried three times before giving up. Ethan's veins are so scarred it was not possible to get in a new line.

Now this tiny boy is down to just one viable IV site. This means they have to discontinue the antibiotics, as these can't be mixed with other medications through a single IV line.

The doctor is also concerned Ethan's air passageway is collapsing. The throat swelling is so bad she couldn't get the vent tube re-inserted—forcing her to put Ethan back on CPAP again.

It seems we're forever taking one step forward and three steps back.

A idan is apparently not ready to go home. This morning he had blood in his stool. Discharge is placed on hold.

The doctors aren't sure what's causing this. X-rays and lab work are ordered. We'll have to wait to see if these will give us a clue as to the cause.

In the meantime, we're back to wearing isolation gear. I'm not worried, just perturbed at having to wear the isolation gown, mask, and gloves again. I never did like these things. They're so hot and confining. Nana's not too thrilled either—says wearing them triggers constant hot flashes.

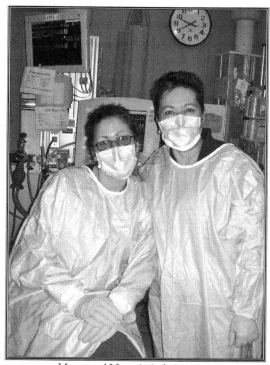

Mama and Nana in isolation gowns

Tuesday, December 19, 2006
NICU Day 72

As I push through the double doors to enter the NICU floor this morning, I can see down the long empty hallway into the boys' room. Dr. Lim and Dr. Placket are standing side-by-side staring into Ethan's isolette. My heart stops and only starts again when they turn around and I see their faces. They both have big smiles!

"Ethan is doing well on CPAP," Dr. Placket says in a celebratory tone. "His blood gas this morning looks beautiful. It's just possible this little one has finally made it off the vent."

I wish I had my camera to take a picture of these two doctors. They are positively beaming.

***

Aidan has blood in his stool yet again. We're still waiting on yesterday's lab work to find out why. Could he be lactose intolerant? Is this the sign of a serious bacterium? Ulcer? NEC? Have I been so preoccupied with Ethan that I missed a sign of trouble for my precious Aidan?

Nana tells me to quit obsessing.

"Welcome to parenthood," she says with a laugh. "You'll have a lifetime to doubt and second guess yourself."

We head upstairs to the hospital café for a fast cup of coffee. Enjoying our break from the NICU, we joke saying we need to invent a microchip that can be implanted in each baby to tell us instantly what is wrong. If microchips can be used in automobiles to monitor mechanical systems, why can't we invent one to monitor human systems? We'd just plug the baby into a computer, and out would pop a printout itemizing what's wrong. No more waiting on lab results!

***

It is noon and Aidan's bloody stool continues. Our attention has been so riveted on Ethan this past week—the bloody stool serves as reminder Aidan is still a micro-preemie with health issues too.

While Aidan sleeps peacefully, I turn to watch the respiratory therapist adjusts Ethan's CPAP pressure down one full notch. Every change in oxygen settings is a sign that Ethan's lungs are getting stronger. Moving down a full setting is an exciting reassurance Ethan may have indeed turned a corner.

CPAP is less invasive than the vent, but Ethan wants it made perfectly clear he *does not like* the mask. The respiratory therapists have tried every trick they know to make it more comfortable, but tiny Ethan still uses every ounce of his energy to fidget and pull at the mask.

Today the respiratory therapist has something exciting to share—he found a new mask style. This one has nose prongs and covers a smaller amount of the face. However, Ethan refuses to wear this one as well. What a sight to see; a therapist trying to wrestle a three-pound baby into a facemask...and lose!

Wednesday, December 20, 2006
NICU Day 73

The region is still recovering from the windstorm and the affects of the massive power outage. Staffing continues to be in turmoil as nurses are shifted from floor to floor to get the proper nurse-patient coverage.

The NICU is full of babies and I help where I can with non-patient chores. Being needed at the NICU softens the disappointment of losing the entire supply of breast milk stored in our thawed-out freezer at home.

Papa made it in again today. I don't know how he is able to navigate the debris-filled roads, but he has not missed a single day since the boys were born. Everyday he is here to talk with the twins, tell stories, and promise fun adventures. I know the babies recognize their Papa's voice.

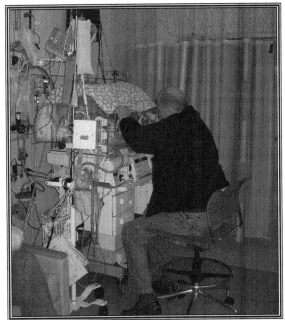

Papa talking to Ethan – Blanket over the isolette blocks the bright lights

***

We're in a repetitive routine at the NICU. When Aidan drops his breathing rate and desats, the alarm flashes a yellow light and buzzes a soft '*beep-beep-beep*.' I reach into his crib to rub his back. This stimulation helps Aidan remember to take a deep breath to raise his oxygen level.

Ethan drops his breathing rate and sets off his alarms. Papa reaches through the isolette armhole and gently strokes Ethan's feet to trigger a deeper breath.

Papa and I spend the long days at the NICU, each stationed next to one of the twins. When the desat alarm beeps, we automatically reach in and touch the baby to remind them to breathe deeply. This happens so often we don't even consciously think about it anymore.

In the NICU, the soft beeps of warning alarms ring constantly. The alarms beep when the boys' IVs need to be changed. The alarms beep when the blood oxygen level drops. They ring loudly when the blood pressure, heart rate, or breathing patterns change up or down more than a couple points.

We memorized the language of the alarm sounds—they are the everyday sounds of our NICU world. I can sleep through a blaring alarm clock, but let there be a soft beep of a monitor alarm and I am instantly alert.

Thursday, December 21, 2006
NICU Day 74

Nurse Julie bought each of the boys a Christmas present—a pacifier called a WubbaNub. This item is so popular apparently there's even a web site dedicated to it. The pacifier comes with a soft stuffed animal attached at one end. Aidan's is a yellow duck and Ethan's is a green frog. As a new mom I need to get up to speed with the latest in baby products—a chore I would have enjoyed under other circumstances.

This gift reminds me, I haven't bought anything for the nurses. In fact, I haven't prepared for Christmas at all. I am usually the one who dives into planning family events and decorating for the holidays. There are only three days left before Christmas and I haven't done a single thing.

***

One of my chores before Aidan is discharged is to find a pediatrician. The NICU staff recommends Dr. Clausen. His expertise for high-risk kids is recognized nationally, and he has patients all across the region.

I call his office to set up Aidan as a new patient.

The office receptionist lectures me; "We only take newborns. Since Aidan is 74 days old we do not consider him to be a newborn."

"He may be 74 days old," I say, "but he is so premature he's not even to his due date yet. Why, he hasn't even been discharged from the hospital!"

The receptionist doesn't understand and she hands the phone over to the head nurse.

When the nurse comes on the line she says with warm enthusiasm, "Yes indeed! We are expecting Aidan. Dr. Clausen is well aware of the twins, as Dr. Placket is keeping him informed of their progress. We look forward to seeing your famous micro-preemies."

Her words give me pause. There's that tag line again, "...*famous micro-preemies.*"

***

By this afternoon Aidan's bloody stool is diagnosed as colitis due to bacteria.

We're still in isolation lock-down with gowns, gloves, and masks to keep from spreading the bacteria.

Discharge before Christmas is now firmly out of the question.

***

For the past four days Ethan has not had a single day with adequate weight gain and the doctors are concerned.

"Ethan's system can't tolerate any more delays in growth," Dr. Lim says. "Preemies need to gain at the rate of 40 to 45 grams each day. Ethan barely gains 10 grams a day. Some days he even loses weight."

Ethan's formula calories are bumped up from 27 to 30 by adding NTT oral fat. This is easily absorbed and also adds protein. This custom blend of calories is rather difficult to calculate—so the nurses re-check the complex prescription multiple times to be sure they mix the formula correctly.

There is also concern with bone density and Ethan's low calcium rating. The last trimester of a pregnancy is when the fetus would normally lay down bone mass—but my boys missed their entire third trimester.

One more thing for the journal; I learn a new diagnosis today for Ethan. He has rickets—meaning his bones are soft and prone to breaking.

***

Justin arrives home before I do. He calls to say the electricity is finally on. The broken skylight window has been repaired, and the damp carpets can dry out now that we have restored heat. Normalcy returns to our home.

The garage freezer was filled with over a hundred bottles of frozen breast milk. I will have the sad chore of throwing this milk away. Every three hours around the clock, 24-hours each day, pumping breast milk since the boys were born—and it's all gone.

Damn.

Today the boys had their first Respiratory Syncytial Virus (RSV)[24] immunization. This vaccine is reserved for high-risk babies to protect them from a highly infectious virus that hits hard and can be life threatening.

The vaccine can help—unfortunately the injection needs to be repeated monthly during the RSV season, which generally runs from October through March.

This is incredibly expensive—as the vaccines cost $2,000 each! Multiply for twins, repeat monthly during the six-month long RSV season, and you get a bill for $24,000.

Guess what—this vaccine is *specifically excluded* by my medical insurance. I have a comprehensive health policy; shouldn't that mean it covers vaccines?

Further reading on the Internet shows countries such as Canada, Germany, Italy, Israel, and even India; supply this vaccine to high-risk babies. To my dismay, I find out this is not the case here in the states. Whether you get this vaccine is totally dependent on your insurance policy!

Where am I going to get $24,000 cash for these vaccines? The stress of surviving the NICU is amplified with stress for financial survival.

---

[24] RSV can cause severe respiratory problems, including bronchitis and pneumonia in young children, and can be life threatening. Twins, babies with chronic lung disease, or extremely low birth weight babies have an increased risk for RSV disease. According to the Center for Disease Control and Prevention, infants at risk are to be given a monthly RSV vaccine during the syncytial virus season, and the American Academy of Pediatrics recommends this vaccine for all infants under two years of age who have Chronic Lung Disease.

Christmas Day, Monday, December 25, 2006
NICU Day 78

When Justin and I arrive at the NICU, we see little red and white striped caps hung on each isolette. I say a silent *thank you* to the volunteers who spent many hours knitting baby hats.

It is unusually quiet. Suddenly it dawns on me; Ethan no longer cries when someone handles him! He used to cry every time he was touched—but today Ethan is bright and engaged and no fussing.

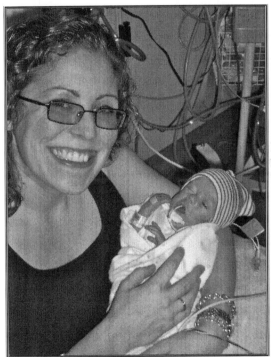

Ethan with no oxygen mask!

Just as we are ready to head out of the NICU for a holiday dinner at Nana and Papa's house, Ethan dislodges his CPAP. In this moment with no mask on his face, Justin snags a photo. There aren't too many photos of Ethan without his oxygen mask.

We delay leaving the hospital for a couple hours to be sure Ethan is okay—resulting in a cold Christmas dinner. Sorry Nana!

Tuesday, December 26, 2006
NICU Day 79

Damn it! A mix up is discovered in Ethan's formula. We are fighting for every gram of weight gain and it took 10 days for someone to notice he was on the wrong formula. This should not be happening.

Ethan was supposed to be on a 30-calorie formula; however the recipe has been mixed wrong. In reality he is still on a 27-calorie mixture.

I am so upset with this. Ethan's lung tissue growth is dependent on his gaining weight and this mess-up happens. My nerves are raw over anything that is out of synch with the plan. I am used to managing a chaotic environment at work—but my nerves can't tolerate a simple mix-up with my son's feeding formula.

***

Yesterday Nurse Julie was able to drop Ethan's oxygen pressure down to a setting of 4.0 and the FiO_2 support down to 34%. His hematocrit unfortunately fell to 29, so an order is place for another blood transfusion (*the 26th one; I am still counting these*). Hopefully this will give Ethan the needed boost in his oxygen saturation levels.

This morning's x-ray shows both of Ethan's lungs are still very cloudy—but they are expanded on all sides. The best news of all; he has been on the nasal cannula all day!

My attitude rises with Ethan's progress—but this is a short-lived celebration. By the time I prepare to leave late this evening, Ethan is struggling to keep his oxygen levels up. The dreadful CPAP machine is brought back. My son does not have enough reserve energy to keep up the pace of breathing in and out with just the cannula.

A idan can go home tomorrow! There were times I doubted this day would ever come. The doctors did mention the possibility of discharge, so I shouldn't be surprised—but I did expect more lead-time than 'tomorrow.'

I am not ready! How can I do this? Do I have the right supplies? How will I ever manage?

Thank goodness my family is here to help. Despite my nervousness, I am overjoyed. At last I am bringing one of my sons home.

Tests are underway as part of the discharge process. Aidan passes the hearing test and I am relieved to learn the heavy doses of antibiotics did not harm his hearing.

The car seat test is passed with flying colors. This means our baby can sit upright in the car seat for a specified length of time and still have enough strength in his chest muscles to breathe on his own.

Aidan's original due date was the third of February. Can you imagine that? He'll be coming home from the NICU before his due date.

Just 24 more hours and our son will come home.

Chapter 21 - *Aidan's Day*

"When you look at your life,
the greatest happiness's are family happiness."

Joyce Brothers

Aidan's Day - Friday, December 29, 2006
NICU Day 82

Today Aidan is coming home—a day we will forever celebrate as 'Aidan's Day'. The twins have their shared birthday and each will have their own 'Coming Home Day.'

Hope was missing when we arrived in the NICU three months ago, but hope is with us today. I can now see that the story of my twins' time in the NICU will end well. I am sure they will survive—they will come home.

The day of their birth was a dark time. Love, faith, and support from the medical team, our family, and our friends gave us the hope we needed. And now, I have one boy headed home. I am forever grateful.

The last weight check is taken—a whooping 2498 grams (~5 lb. 8 oz.). As I dress Aidan, staff from all over the hospital stop in to say goodbye. Even the hospital's CEO sees us off.

The room is a swirl of hectic commotion as we bundle up our son. Throughout all this, Ethan is quiet and alert. Papa sits next to his isolette and tells him not to worry—we'll be back tomorrow.

I have mixed emotions as I carry Aidan through the exit doors. I look over my shoulder and glance down the long hallway to our NICU room. I can barely see Ethan lying inside his isolette. All I see is a mass of IVs, feeding tubes, oxygen lines, and monitor wires. Somewhere in that box lies my baby. It is hard to leave. I want Ethan so badly my chest hurts.

My emotions are held in check and my sorrow is softened as soon as I bring Aidan into his new home. Justin and I take turns carrying our son from room to room as we introduce him to his new surroundings, his new bedroom, and his new pets.

Jameson is curious. Wagging his tail in anticipation he drops a tennis ball next to Aidan's infant seat—just in case this baby wants to play a game of fetch.

For the first time in his life, Aidan sleeps at home.

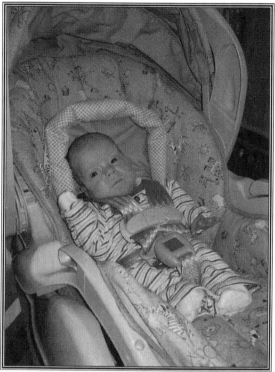

Aidan on discharge day - 3 months old - 5 lbs. 8 oz.

Tuesday, January 2, 2007
NICU Day 86

Today holds a milestone for Ethan. He gets his first oral feeding! Nurse Julie feeds him using a miniature bottle. Ethan choked and sputtered and managed to take 5 cc—about one teaspoon. It is hard for Ethan to get good suction on the nipple because his palate has been altered by the long stint on ventilators. The vent tubing made the roof of his mouth form a high arch and this in turn makes him more prone to choke and gag.

Julie is patient and whispers encouragement to him.

"Don't worry Ethan. You'll get the hang of this eventually."

***

Ethan is strong enough now to move his head from side to side all by himself. He figured out by turning his head in a rocking motion, he could loosen the seal of the CPAP mask. Once there is a break in the seal, Ethan pulls at the tubing to fully dislodge the mask pressure. He is our NICU Houdini Escape Artist—capable of amazing feats for a frail baby.

To thwart Ethan's attempts, the nurse tapes the CPAP tubes to the inside wall of the isolette—running them up the side and across the lid so they dangle directly above Ethan's face—supposedly out of reach of his little hands.

The nurse hasn't even left the room yet and Ethan has already managed to kick his scrawny legs up to the isolette lid where his feet tangle in the CPAP tubing.

Where does this three-pound baby get such a spunky attitude?

***

We have another milestone to celebrate. Ethan is able to keep his body temperature up without the help of the warming isolette. This afternoon he is moved to an open crib. At last, Ethan is out of the enclosed plastic box he has called home for so long.

His new bed is not a regular baby-crib with side rails; rather it is a small open-topped box meant to hold one infant. While it may be meant for a single baby, it is still big enough to hold *both* of my tiny boys.

Normally, siblings aren't allowed into the NICU—but an exception is made for Aidan. When I bring Aidan to the NICU to visit Ethan, I tuck him next to his brother in this open crib. The babies snuggle and fall asleep in each other's arms—it is the sweetest thing I've ever seen.

These brothers are identical twins, but when laying side-by-side it is so apparent Ethan needs substantial catch-up in weight gain.

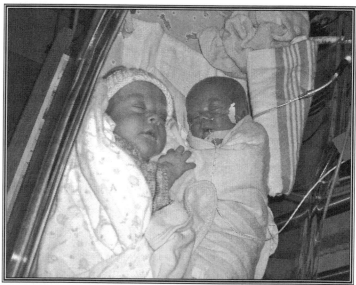

Aidan (5 lbs. 10 oz.) and Ethan on cannula oxygen (4 lbs. 4 oz.)

Thursday, January 4, 2007
NICU Day 88

D r. Lim stops by our NICU room just as Ethan attacks his bottle. He laughs and calls Ethan his little 'Cookie Monster.' I love this nickname and hope Ethan lives up to this by continuing to eat.

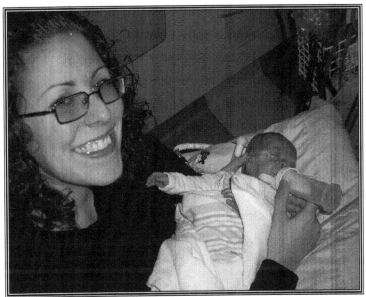

"Cookie Monster" Ethan

Ethan took 25 cc of breast milk by bottle and this little guy did it with a #5 flow rate nipple. No more micropreemie nipples for Ethan. If a larger holed nipple is considered a step up, we will call this a milestone. I am willing to celebrate *anything* as a sign of progress.

Most of the day is just a recycle of prior days. I think we're locked in a *Groundhog's Day* movie; each day is a repeat of the day before.

Friday, January 5, 2007
NICU Day: 89

This morning I pester Dr. Baillie to predict how long before Ethan can come home.

"Ethan needs to gain another 1000 grams," he says. "If he can put on this much weight, his lungs will be strong enough to breathe on his own."

Another 1000 grams? I think this is an impossible goal for a baby who rarely gains more than 10 grams a day.

***

Ethan has rickets. He did not get enough calcium laid down before his preterm birth, so his bones are prone to breaking. To improve the low bone density, Nurse Julie tells me the plan is to add calcium and phosphorous to his diet. The problem is there is no preemie compound for this supplement. Julie has to crush an adult tablet of calcium, mix it with warm water, and push the mixture down Ethan's NG feeding tube.

Unfortunately this compound will set up like cement if it cools to room temperature. The glob of calcium doesn't flow down the nasogastric tube fast enough before it cools and solidifies, plugging up the tube.

Julie removes the feeding tube and tries to salvage the balance of the calcium stuck inside. She looks into the end of the tube and gives it a gentle squeeze. The tube explodes like a cannon—spewing white paste all over. What a mess. There is calcium plastered everywhere.

Wish I had a picture of Julie's silly grin as she stands there with white paste hanging off her eyelashes.

Monday, January 8, 2007
NICU Day 92

I thought once we got a baby home things would improve; but it is so much harder than I ever imagined. Aidan is doing his best to make sure I never get any sleep. His reflux is dreadful. Everything he eats seems to come back up in projectile vomit. All I ever do is wash and feed this baby. I gave up trying to wash and feed myself. There's no time for that.

***

Each morning I bundle up Aidan for the trip back to the NICU where we spend the day with Ethan. I am so glad they made an exception to allow Aidan to visit.

Today I watch as the ultrasound equipment is wheeled in to check on Ethan's brain bleed.

As the tech rolls the scanner out of the room, Dr. Baillie explains the results.

"The scan shows the major blood clot in the brain is resolving. The clots in the ventricles have clumped together and are reducing in size as Ethan's body works to dissolve each clot. I think it might be another three or four weeks before this is totally resolved."

"The ventricle size is the same—no more swelling. Once the clots are gone, the extra fluid that built up in the ventricle will be re-absorbed. The clots in the brain tissue that formed into PVL cysts are just slightly larger than the original blood clot."

He wraps up flashing a quick thumbs-up gesture. "In short, I am optimistic all of this will wrap-up with no major side effects."

Got to love this prediction!

Chapter 22 - *Eye Trouble*

"Anyone can hold the helm when the sea is calm."

Unknown

Wednesday, January 10, 2007
NICU Day 94

The day starts just like all the repetitious days that went before. Ethan continues to alternate between the cannula and CPAP oxygen support. He tires easily and burns so many calories just breathing that he doesn't gain any weight. Three months old and he only weighs 4 lb. 14 oz.

This afternoon the repetition continues with yet one more ROP eye test. This particular test has become so frequent and routine I don't even give it a second thought.

How wrong I was. Today's ROP test is a disaster!

Ethan moved rapidly to Stage III ROP in both eyes. The speed of deterioration is of great concern and the ophthalmologist says Ethan needs eye surgery. He really frightens me when he says the surgery must be done *immediately*, and adds emphasis by slapping one hand against his open palm.

"Can we wait to see if this resolves itself?" I ask.

"If we gamble and hold off on surgery, you risk having a blind baby," the doctor quickly replies. "If the ROP progresses any further Ethan will be blind. When ROP gets to Stage IV nothing can be done to reverse the vision lost."

"We have to move quickly. At Stage III, this little guy has already lost some vision. He needs surgery right away to prevent any more vision lost."

The threat of blindness is shocking. I try to digest what the doctor says about the surgery. My impression from this hurried discussion is *this surgery is not life threatening* and *it is always successful.* Or maybe that's what I wanted to hear.

As the doctor prepares orders to move Ethan for immediate surgery, I rummage through my tote bag for my cell phone to call Justin with the news.

Things are moving fast. Ethan is transferred to Mercy Hospital this morning and surgery is set to occur immediately upon his arrival. Papa is taking care of Aidan at home and poor Justin is stuck handling a key customer account. When you're trying to hang on to every potential customer, there aren't many choices about work schedules.

The transport team has Ethan en route under a red flashing emergency light. 'Lead-foot' Nana drives me to Mercy Hospital—arriving almost at the same time as Ethan.

They have taken my baby straight into the operating room. Dr. Englund stops just outside of the OR for a quick explanation of the procedure and the predicted outcome. He's in a hurry, so he rattles off a list of stats very quickly, saying…

60% chance of success *(we expected 90%);*

40% chance this will not work and Ethan will be blind *(we thought there was virtually no chance of blindness if surgery was done right away)*;

Surgery itself will cause some vision loss *(we expected no additional loss of vision)*;

Surgery either works or it doesn't. It can't be done again *(we thought surgery could be repeated until successful)*.

I am overwhelmed with these statistics, as they don't match my expectations—but I can't think of any more questions.

Dr. Englund quickly turns on his heels and rushes into the OR.

Nana and I begin the long wait.

We sit in the waiting room for hours—oblivious to all that come and go. I don't think I breathed the entire time. This is petrifying. I just keep thinking *40% chance of complete blindness.*

How do I deal with a blind baby?

What will it be like for one twin to see and the other not?

What if he's blind *and* has cerebral palsy?

And in the back of my mind I recall the doctors' warnings that Ethan is at risk for severe hearing loss due to the heavy doses of antibiotics.

It seems they keep taking bits and pieces of Ethan.

Will there be anything left?

***

More than three hours later, Dr. Englund comes into the waiting area with his facemask dangling loose around his neck and wearing a huge grin. As he walks towards me, he flashes a double thumbs-up gesture.

I can breathe again.

The surgery is described as successful. He explains Ethan's vision impairment will be limited to a loss of peripheral vision in both eyes. This is something Ethan will probably not be consciously aware of, as he will never know what it would be like to have side-vision.

Dr. Englund lowers his large frame onto the tiny waiting room chair. The big smile is gone now; he is all business. He speaks softly saying, "Ethan's eyes are doing well, but he's still on the ventilator. The settings are rather high post surgery and I am a bit concerned as to why he needs so much oxygen support."

We've dealt with ventilator issues for so long this does not surprise us. Hearing what we consider to be good news on the outcome of the eye surgery, Nana takes off to relieve Papa. He's been babysitting Aidan solo and surely must be exhausted by now.

Justin gets to the hospital as soon as he can after work. From his jobsite at a town 50 miles south of here, the commute—plus rush hour congestion—would normally keep him on the roads well over two hours; but he navigates in record time driving illegally in the carpool lane.

The two of us stay very late. We would have spent the night, but there were no sleeping rooms available. The sleeping cubbies filled up early today, as many parents are stranded here due to the snow and ice storm that blew in this morning.

It is midnight when we head home and ours is the only car on the road.

I sure don't look forward to tomorrow's long drive back through all this snow and ice.

D r. Seaton, the Chief of Medicine for the NICU stops by the room to personally check on Ethan. She remembers us from our last stay here and even asks how Aidan is doing.

Recalling I like to hear details of the medical plan, she takes her time talking with me. I learn that an echocardiogram has been ordered for this afternoon to measure Ethan's heart chamber size.

The doctors here (and at Mission Valley) continue to focus on Ethan's heart. It's as if they expect to find cardiac issues. None are found—not yet anyway.

"It's important to get Ethan's lungs back to the pre-surgery baseline by tomorrow morning," explains Dr. Seaton. "That's when I have the pediatric pulmonologist coming to look at Ethan's lungs and trachea."

I didn't know she called in a sub-specialist to evaluate Ethan. I just want to go back to Mission Valley; but as long as the pulmonologist is coming, I hope he will figure out why so much oxygen support is needed so we can get out of here.

The pediatric pulmonologist has just arrived. He has to use two hands to heft up Ethan's overflowing medical chart.

"This little guy's oxygen saturation levels are only in the upper 60's," he says. "These numbers are indicative of poor gas exchange and Ethan's shallow breathing is not optimal. He will not grow if this much energy is taken up just trying to breathe."

The doctor is silent for a brief moment, then adds; "This chronic lung disease is out of control."

While pacing the room he describes the issues. "X-ray films show considerable scar tissue. I don't know how this baby is able to survive without a trach. His lungs may eventually heal themselves, but if the healing is too slow this baby will need a trach."

We've heard this trach discussion before, so Nana and I don't ask questions on this topic.

The doctor slides a roller-wheeled chair from the computer table over towards me. Straddling the chair he says, "I am concerned Ethan may have a floppy trachea—meaning the walls of the trachea collapse."

"Ethan's lungs are not fully recruited—especially the upper right lobe which is severely compromised. The stats show CO_2 hovering in the 60's. I'd like to continue to use CPAP to keep the trachea open after he comes off the vent."

And to make sure we understand the seriousness of this number he adds; "CO_2 at this level is a sign of respiratory failure."

There are so many questions to ask and he takes his time and answers them all patiently and clearly.

I ask him about the floppy trachea.

"This is called trachea malaise. It occurs when the baby's windpipe clamps down on the vent tube. Once the vent tube is removed, the trachea has a tendency to flop closed. Ethan has the largest tube diameter I've ever seen in a baby this small. This is going to be problematic when the tube is eventually removed, as it has caused considerable tracheal stretching."

"The pressure from CPAP will help keep the windpipe open after the tube is removed. It can be nine to 12 months before the trachea grows strong enough not to collapse. And you need to know the longer a baby is on the vent, the more long-term the lung damage."

The doctor stands up and walks over to the crib. He takes out a stethoscope and listens to Ethan's lungs. Right away the doctor's face lights up with a big smile.

Looking up he says, "I hear strong air movement—Ethan is not breathing overly hard. The lungs sound crackly, but not wheezy. I studied Ethan's charts in great detail before coming into this room. The counsel I just gave you was based on his charts. I must tell you, I am a bit surprised at the spunk of this tiny baby."

The doctor is again pacing the room and his speech is as fast as his walk.

"The next step is to put Ethan on another series of prednisone. Long steroid use can cause heart problems, so we will watch the heart closely. If Ethan has high blood pressure in one chamber of the heart, this can be problematic—and chronic lung disease is a major contributor to heart problems."

I ask him to summarize his opinion now that he has both read Ethan's charts and listened to his lungs.

He looks at me for several long seconds—and slowly drawing out each word for me, he says; "Your baby's lungs are very damaged."

Monday, January 15, 2007
NICU Day 99

At morning rounds we hear that Ethan's ventilator has another leak around the tubing and the doctors can't get an accurate blood gas reading. This might be why his oxygen and CO_2 levels are not stabilizing.

The doctors are considering intubation with a 4.0 mm tube to solve the air leak. They caution this dramatic solution is not without risks, as they have never had a tube this large in a baby so small. I am told the larger tube will continue to stretch and damage Ethan's trachea. This is a significant move, so the medical team is conferring with sub-specialists before proceeding.

***

Ethan's eyes look scratchy and appear more swollen than yesterday. I bathe them with a warm washcloth to wipe off the gunk and to sooth them.

While I tend to my son, the nurses come and go—always in a rush to complete a procedure in the room and move on. They bustle about adjusting the machines, but never once do they stop to offer comfort to this baby. They never really look at Ethan—their eyes are too busy scanning the monitors and recording stats. I wonder if they even know his name.

As I lean over the crib to bathe Ethan's crusty eyes, I hear the wet sounds of his breathing. Even with the background noise of the NICU, I can hear his raspy and wet gurgles. It has always been like this. I have never heard my son take a normal breath. Ethan's soft shallow breathing is always accompanied with the rattle of compromised lungs. Oh how I wish I could fill his lungs with air and breathe for him.

Yesterday evening the doctors decided the larger vent tube was the best solution to resolve the air leak. Ethan is re-intubated with a 4.0 mm tube. This eliminated the leak for now and oxygen vent settings are dropping nicely.

Dr. Englund, the eye surgeon is here to check on his patient. He uses a scope to peer into Ethan's eyes. After a long minute, he turns to face me wearing a big smile.

"Ethan's eyes look really good post-op. I see the ROP ridge is regressing. This is exactly how we want it to look at this point. I am confident we got it all—but Ethan will need to be re-tested in a month or so to verify the ROP progression has stopped."

I like the prediction he got it all—but I worry just a bit when he says Ethan has to be monitored to be sure the ROP doesn't return.

***

This morning we have the worst dayshift nurse ever. I refer to her as Nurse No-No.

She constantly turns up Ethan's vent to higher and higher settings. This is counter to our goal of *decreasing* oxygen support.

I tell her, "He doesn't need the oxygen pressure increased every time he desats. Just touch him on his feet. This touch will remind him to breathe deeper and he will come out of the desat on his own."

To show her, I gently touch Ethan's feet.

"See, like this," I say. "He will come back up on his own with just a little rub and then…"

Nurse No-No cuts me off saying, "No. No. I can't be doing this. There are other sick babies in my charge and I don't have time for this."

My hackles rise, but I am controlled and speak softly as I repeat; "When the oximeter alarm beeps, he just needs a gentle reminder to breathe. Rub his feet and he will remember to take a deeper breath."

She shoots back saying, "Look, I said *no*. I can't keep running in here every time he triggers the alarm."

The stress continues to chip away at me.

I can't take this much longer.

***

It has been a long day of ups and downs, and by evening it's mostly down. Ethan is constantly desatting as his blood oxygen level drops precipitously. All of his IV lines have blown. He has no veins that can hold an IV for more than a day. The docs put him on oral sedatives as they try to stabilize stats.

As I post today's date in my journal, I realize this is our 100th day in intensive care.

There is something defeating in this milestone.

Thursday, January 18, 2007
NICU Day 102

Ethan is quite agitated. Something is not right. It takes a couple minutes until I track down two nurses standing at the end of the hall. I tell them something is bothering my son. They don't really listen. From their expressions I can tell they are preoccupied and not really listening. They seem to have dismissed my observation as unimportant even before I finish describing it.

At morning rounds I mention it again; Ethan seems unusually agitated. The attending doctor nods his head at my comments as if agreeing; but the discussion ends abruptly mid-sentence when a series of red alarms blare simultaneously from two nearby rooms. As the doctors split off in two directions, my question hangs in the air unanswered.

I head back to Ethan's room and find a nurse has come to hang a dose of prednisone.

Why is she starting prednisone now?

According to my notes, the prednisone was supposed to have started 12 hours ago. The nurse shrugs saying the order was overlooked and they just now caught it.

Before she leaves the room, I point out to her that Ethan seems to be more agitated than usual.

"Look at him," I say. "See how he grimaces each time he tries to inhale? Can you get one of the doctors to come in here?"

The nurse doesn't even look at Ethan; rather with a reflexive glance she looks at his array of monitors—none of which show any sign of trouble. She nods absently, but I get the impression there won't be any urgency to find a doctor.

Two hours later a doctor stops by and the mystery of Ethan's agitated is solved.

"I just read Ethan's morning x-ray," the doctor says, "and it shows another collapse in his right lung."

No wonder Ethan has been agitated all morning!

I told the nurses he was distressed. I told the doctors at morning rounds Ethan was agitated more than normal. They don't listen to the parent. I am the one sitting by my baby's bedside day after day; *I know* when he is agitated.

If these doctors did rounds at the bedside rather than way off at the Nurses' Station, and if they actually looked at the baby…well, maybe they'd see this for themselves.

The doctors at Mission Valley would have listened to me. They would have tried to find out why Ethan was agitated. But I just hold my thoughts, thank the doctor for the information, and calmly ask how he plans to treat this latest lung collapse.

***

The pulmonologist delivered his evaluation to the medical team at rounds, but he stops by our room this afternoon to personally update me.

"After careful consideration I think Ethan will need a trach eventually to help with breathing. This can't happen just yet—he is far too fragile to survive surgery. First, Ethan needs to go back to Mission Valley to grow more lung tissue. When he is strong enough, we'll bring him back to Mercy for trach surgery."

"Don't worry," he adds. "A trach is not as bad as it sounds. Most kids flourish and grow on a trach."

I am not so sure I agree that kids *flourish* with a trach. I dealt with kids on trachs when I interned in Special Education during my university studies. I know what's in store for children tethered to an oxygen machine for years.

At least we're going back to Mission Valley. I'd rather the trach decision be made by doctors who know Ethan.

I am tired.

I just want to get Ethan out of here.

Chapter 23 - *"Sweet Child of Mine"*

"We need hope to survive,
but it is with laughter we live."

Michele M. Kemper

Saturday, January 20, 2007
NICU Day 104

Ethan is transferred back to Mission Valley this afternoon. Dr. Lim is waiting as we arrive and I can tell right away he is not happy with Ethan's condition. I don't hear the doctor say anything outright negative, but it's apparent he is not happy with Ethan's lungs.

After five days at Mercy, Ethan's lungs once again are in worse shape than when he left Mission. Transferring back and forth between hospitals may solve surgical issues, but it is hell on lung recovery.

Ethan is agitated when he arrives—he needs to be fed! Mercy held the morning feedings while pending the transfer. This medical team should have adjusted the feeding schedule *before* the transfer so this baby could eat.

Now Ethan is crying so hard he is vomiting up any food he is given. The doctors have to give him a dose of morphine to relax him so he won't over-exert his lungs.

I am so mad at Mercy Hospital—this is inexcusable. Had the medical team viewed Ethan's needs as central to the transfer plan, they would have adjusted his feeding schedule ahead of time.

***

Mission Valley's team completes their workup and my poor baby has to endure more pokes for blood draws. The lab work shows the hematocrit reading is low and a blood transfusion (*his 27th*) is ordered for tonight.

With all the commotion from the transfer and blood draws, Ethan is upset. I try to comfort him, but he is too tired and too hungry to be calmed.

Finally it dawns on me what to do. I lay Aidan in the open-air crib with his brother and his presence calms

Ethan. They stare into each other's face—as if to wonder where the heck their brother has been for so long. The boys snuggle their tiny bodies together and immediately fall asleep.

***

After a long day at the NICU, Justin and I head home with Aidan. Just as we climb into bed, the phone rings. The ring tone is set to identify the caller, so I know it is the NICU when I hear *Sweet Child of Mine* (by Guns N Roses).

My heart freezes as Justin picks up the phone and puts it on speaker.

The laughter in Dr. Lim's voice comes clearly across the line. "Ethan pulled out his vent tube and is doing very well without it!"

I smile as I hear him joke; "You need to have a talk with your son about his attitude on ventilators."

What a lovely phone call. Imagine a doctor calling to say everything is okay. Dr. Lim is the only one to do this and I treasure this call.

I can sleep at last. Well, sleep for an hour anyway until Aidan wakes for one of his many nighttime feedings.

Sunday, January 21, 2007
NICU Day 105

The NICU room needs to be decorated. This will be our home for some time yet to come and I decide it needs to looks like a baby lives here. I bring in a portable baby swing for Aidan to use, and a mobile for Ethan's crib so he has something to look at besides IV lines.

The double-seat stroller is piled high with extra baby gear, and Aidan is tucked in there somewhere along with the tote bags. As I come around the corner pushing the stroller towards Ethan's room, I can hear Nurse Julie's voice. She is telling Ethan how happy everyone is to have him home again.

Julie looks up and smiles as I push the double-long stroller into the private room. She gives details of Ethan's nighttime stats, noting that feeds were increased to 43 cc and morphine and sedatives have been discontinued. For now, the plan is to use steroids and diuretics to try to pull fluids out of the lungs.

I look at Julie and give a slight nod of my head in the direction of Dr. Lim. The doctor, perched with perfect posture on the stool next to Ethan's crib, makes minute adjustments to the oxygen machine.

Julie answers my unasked question as she silently mouths the words, "He spent all night here."

Apparently after Dr. Lim called us last night, he stayed the entire evening with Ethan to keep an eye on things. He must be exhausted—yet he does not show it. I think this man could walk through hell and come out looking impeccably groomed and calm. Come to think of it, he has walked through hell more than once taking care of my babies!

Monday, January 22, 2007
NICU Day 106

Aidan comes with me every day to visit his brother. I prop him in the baby swing where he holds court with all who come to the room. Mostly he prefers to be held; and there is never a shortage of arms that want to hold Aidan. Usually it is Nana and Papa, but just as often it is one of the doctors or nurses who stop by and hold Aidan.

During the day the babies co-bed. They talk to each other with cooing sounds, and squirm until their heads are pressed together. They look so content. I wish I could crawl into the crib with them.

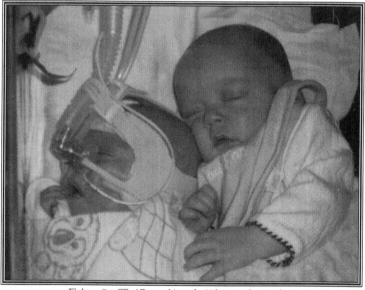

Ethan (in CPAP mask) and Aidan - asleep at last

***

Dr. Lim gives the morning status update. "CPAP settings were at 8.0," he says, "but Ethan is doing so well I was able to turn the pressure down two full settings to 6.0. The CO_2 levels dropped to 52 (closer to the target of 35 to 40), and FiO_2 is 30—all lower than any time at Mercy."

"Ethan's blood oxygen saturations continue to be stable, and the numbers are staying up where they should be. Also, Ethan's tracheal malaise is mild and not something to worry about at this time. The issue we need to be concerned with right now is his lungs."

Dr. Lim pauses briefly, taking a quick glance at his pager that just buzzed. Deleting the message on the screen, he continues.

"The lung sounds today are good, and Ethan is not struggling to breathe. He is doing so much better now that he is off the ventilator."

Mercy Hospital's plan was to keep Ethan on a vent, but Dr. Lim says he could have told them this would not work. Ethan hates the ventilator even more than he hates CPAP! When Ethan is on the vent he struggles constantly and over-taxes his lungs—which totally defeats the purpose.

Just think. Two days ago the prediction was Ethan would need a trach.

I wonder…are we out of the woods yet?

***

At home the nighttime routine is crazy. Aidan needs to eat every three hours and I need to pump at the same time. When Aidan starts to wake, Justin runs to heat the bottle while I get Aidan's diaper changed.

My tiny son is still not strong enough to nurse, so he has to take breast milk by bottle. While Justin feeds Aidan, I get hooked up to the breast pump.

We usually watch the Discovery Channel during this 45-minute routine. There isn't much else on TV in the middle of the night.

Tonight's show is about bats. Jeez—from baby poop to bat guano!

Tuesday, January 23, 2007
NICU Day 107

D r. Placket thinks Ethan might have an inguinal hernia. One testicle has dropped and one did not. There has been no stool in 24 hours and this adds a layer of concern—especially if this is because of the suspected hernia.

I'm told hernias are extremely common in preemies. If Ethan has one, he'll need surgery. As long as his bowels are working there are no worries for now. This surgery can wait until he is much stronger.

The conversation with Dr. Placket shifts to selecting a pediatrician for Ethan. I tell him we are set up with Dr. Clausen—the same doctor we picked for Aidan. As we chat about pediatricians, Mom happens to mentions Dr. Roger Malet was my pediatrician back in the late '70's and '80's.

Dr. Placket's eyes open wide. "Dr. Malet was my partner at the Avondale Pediatric Clinic during that time!"

No wonder Mom had the nagging thought she had met Dr. Placket some time in the past. He was one of the pediatricians covering my own well-baby check-ups three decades earlier!

Wednesday, January 24, 2007
NICU Day 108

My career has always been so important to me. I have a financial securities Registered Rep license—which places me on the advanced track with my employer. I have seven years with this company and I was excited to take on additional responsibilities just before everything came to a screeching halt with the boys' premature delivery.

My work has been center-stage for so long. I am a bit surprised I have not given much thought to my job over the past three months while on leave. It is as if my work life is frozen in another world I will re-enter later.

Sometimes I fantasize my boss reaches out to tell me not to worry. I wish he'd say *everything will be here waiting for you.* But these words never come.

Tonight I find a voicemail on my answering machine from my boss. I am shocked at his words, and play the message over to be sure I am hearing it correctly. He sounds angry and says I am "…milking this family leave thing far too long…" and wants to know "…when the hell I plan to get back to work."

His words are disguised as if they are a joke by adding a forced laugh as an afterthought just before abruptly hanging up.

When I started my leave of absence it was agreed this would be time off without pay until the pre-arranged return date of April 16.

Why is he calling now?

Will I lose my job too?

Thursday, January 25, 2007
NICU Day 109

Nurse Modra rotates back to the NICU and specifically asks to be assigned to Ethan. It's good to have her back. She's an experienced nurse, but even Modra has a hard time keeping the CPAP mask on Ethan. Equipment designed for very small babies is still too big for him. Ethan is so tiny the oxygen mask slip off his micro-preemie size face.

Modra enlists the respiratory therapist to help find a way to hold the mask in place. While these two are fussing with the facemask, I make a dash to the café for a cup of coffee.

When I return, I chuckle at the sight that greets me. The respiratory therapist is sitting on the floor with a surgical kit of needles and brightly colored suture thread as he hand-sews the straps of the cap to fit Ethan. He even embroiders a little "E" with green thread. This handy stitching reduces the CPAP mask to a miniature size so it won't slide around so easily on Ethan's head.

***

I'm told Nurse Practitioner Josephine will be here this afternoon as she is again assigned a rotation with this hospital. A phenomenally talented practitioner and such a great personality—I'm looking forward seeing her. Just five minutes with Josephine and everyone will be smiling at her witty comments. Her upbeat spirit provides a welcomed relief in a place with so much sadness.

It has been a long time since Josephine saw Ethan, so Nurse Joan and I decide to play the 'Switch the Identical Twin' trick on her.

We put Aidan into the crib, and I hold Ethan tethered to his oxygen tank while hiding behind the privacy screen.

We hope Josephine will mistake the much bigger Aidan for his identical twin—only Josephine visits the patient rooms in *reverse order* today and our short-lived trick falls flat. We enjoyed our little joke—even though no one else saw it.

Nana arrives at the NICU after this stunt and she knows right away what the problem is; too much stress and not enough laughter in my day.

As Nana and I head to the cafeteria for a bowl of soup, she continues to brighten my day with a series of funny stories. For a few minutes I laugh and feel refreshed.

Nana's face brightens as she shares a wild idea; "What this hospital needs is a visit from Ellen (DeGeneres)! If anyone can brighten the day, she can."

When this nightmare is over, Nana says she'll invite Ellen to come have coffee with us! Silly as all this sounds, the banter makes me smile. I sorely needed this break.

Maybe I should warn Ellen? My mother can be pretty determined!

Chapter 24 - *It Cost What?*

*"Choosing between financial solvency
and medical care for your child
should never be a choice forced on a family."*

Michele M. Kemper

Monday, January 29, 2007
NICU Day 113

odern medicine can perform miracles. These miracles however are expensive. Health care costs consume a far larger portion of our gross domestic product than they do for any other developed nation in the world. No wonder health care is part of our national debate.

According to a current news article I found on CNN's website, the average cost for a premature baby for the first year of life is about $49,000. By contrast, they say a newborn without complications costs $4,551.

The article goes on to explain that the majority of this expense is covered by medical insurance and the parents are left to pay out-of-pocket in the range of $2,000.

This is a fantasy world!

I'd sure like to talk to the researcher who wrote this article and find out where the hell he got those numbers.

Let me tell you the real story.

Bills of $500,000 for a preterm baby are not unusual for the NICU; and bills of more than *a million dollars* are not unheard of for a micro-preemie. Our twin micro-preemies will rack up medical bills in just the first 24 months of their life totaling over $2.1 million. And it does not end here. Like many parents with critically or chronically ill kids, we will be overwhelmed with ongoing medical bills for years to come.

What family can afford these enormous sums without insurance? Even with a robust health insurance plan, families typically find their insurance contract has gaps in coverage that leave large balances to pay.

Virtually all private insurance takes the form of some version of managed care. This means, before treatments can be given, the need for the treatment must be justified. Most insurance policies have a list of items they *pre-*

determined would simply not be covered—regardless of their justification.

Our so-called comprehensive insurance policy has several of these exclusions. I had no idea these gaps existed. I was told at annual all-employee meetings just how wonderfully rich our benefit package was. And I received a summary handbook of the medical plan with two points highlighted in bold font:

- No lifetime maximum payout cap
- Annual out-of-pocket $1,500/person or $3,000/family

This is misleading! I now find out this medical policy *specifically excludes* certain treatments used for premature babies—meaning these bills will not be covered. The exclusions require us to pay a whole lot more than $3,000 per family. The gaps in coverage will leave us with balances due totaling four times our annual salary in the first year alone. I am certain we will be forced into bankruptcy before this is over.

With a little bit of research and a few pushy phone calls, I am able to get through to a senior executive at my insurance company. He thinks I am calling to interview him in regards an article I'm writing on medical insurance. This is a frank discussion. He tells me it is a common practice for insurance companies to exclude certain conditions that generate a high cost in medical bills. Without these exclusions, insurance premiums would be outrageous.

"We can't cover everything," he says. "We need to find ways to keep insurance affordable. Most people would consider it unfair to be charged for a medical event that would probably never happen to them or their family."

I am speechless with this inane logic. Heart surgery, kidney dialysis, chemotherapy, and transplants—these life-saving and expensive treatments are covered by my policy, yet it does not cover certain treatments for a preterm baby? Is that because parents of preemies are too preoccupied to form a lobby to force coverage by insurance companies?

***

Since my insurance policy won't pay all the medical expenses, we ask the hospital to assign us a case manager. I need help to sort out how we are to pay the growing hospital bills.

They send us a social worker that looks to be 18 years old. Okay, this is a bit of an exaggeration, but she is young and so inexperienced.

"Do you spend more than you earn?' she asks. "Are you using a credit card for everyday purchases?"

She flips open a notebook and reads from a list of 'yes' or 'no' counseling questions.

"Are your savings inadequate or nonexistent? Do you use cash advances on credit cards to pay off other expenses? Are you getting calls from collection agencies? Have you received notices about utility disconnection?"

I am in such surprise at her naiveté my mouth drops open. She misunderstands this as a sign to continue her patronizing and useless lecture.

"You know procrastination can be your worst enemy. Ignoring financial obligations now can lead to even greater problems later. Instead of putting things off, you can talk to your creditors and arrange alternate payment schedules, accepting partial payments, and so on."

I tell her I am well versed in finances being a Registered Representative for a financial services company. Our problem is these medical expenses are well beyond our reach. We already contacted our mortgage company. They won't even talk to us unless we are more than three months in arrears. We have talked with the hospital's billing department and they said if we want a payment plan they can set one up for a maximum of 90 days.

We have one bill for $260,000! I can't pay this off in 90 days. At the rate bills are accumulating, I can't pay these off in 90 years!

The Social Worker seems to pluck a solution out of thin air when she says, "Well, you could get a bank loan to cover the $260,000."

I ignore her advice and inform her, "You can't get a bank loan for a quarter of a million dollars without collateral."

Gritting my teeth, I hurl a shotgun of curt replies.

"The $260,000 is not a fixed number. It is growing by the day. The pharmacy won't fill the order for Aidan's prescription formula unless I pay for it in advance—and this costs me $450 each month. And then there's the RSV vaccine that costs $2,000 every month. Do you realize this vaccine is needed monthly for the entire RSV season that runs from October to March? The prescription formula and the RSV vaccine are *specifically excluded* from my insurance plan, and Medicare won't help after the babies are discharged from the hospital. How do I come up with this much money every month?"

She is not grasping this, but I continue anyway.

"We average three specialist appointments weekly for Aidan—which totals upwards of $350 just for the office visit co-pays each month."

I stop to catch my breath.

"I need $3,000 every month just for Aidan's medical expenses that are not covered by insurance. And, we haven't even talked yet about Ethan's monthly costs when he is discharged!"

She sighs and flips her notebook closed.

I don't think she heard a word I said.

"Well bottom line," she says, "you need to learn to cut your expenses by making lifestyle changes. When you have a sick child, you need to shift your priorities. Going out to dinner a few times a month may no longer be in your budget. You should find it helpful to compare monthly costs against your income, and then eliminate any expenses which aren't completely necessary like switching to generic prescriptions whenever possible. Or you might try dropping the premium channels on your TV. Also, buy your groceries in bulk and take advantage of coupons and store specials."

She is clueless.

I can see the news headline now...*irate mom attacks social worker with notebook*. I'm not even going to tell you where I want to cram that notebook.

***

When I open the mail this evening, I get a big laugh. My insurance company denied all charges incurred more than three days after the boys' birth—citing the charges as "not medically necessary."

I call the insurance company. The idiot claims processor says my plan only covers newborn care for three days of hospitalization after a C-section. She kept telling me I have to submit a doctor's written permission to keep the babies in the hospital longer than three days.

What does she think? I left my babies at the hospital and forgot to take them home with me?

Despite this silly declination, I know the paperwork will get straightened out eventually. However, what am I going to do with the rest of our bills that are piling up? I emptied our savings account, maxed our home equity line, and filled up our credit cards. There is a modest amount of money in our IRA retirement account, and once that is gone there is nothing left.

My mom and dad step in and give us money to cover our basic living expenses, but I don't know how we'll pay down all these medical bills.

How do other parents of critically ill babies do this? How does one recover from a hit like this?

Everywhere I turn for financial help I am turned away as 'not eligible' because my husband and I are employed, our mortgage is not past due, and I have private health insurance. I have everything to lose and it looks like I will lose it all—house, savings, retirement...even my car.

I refuse to worry about money now. I can't worry about something that I can't solve. It takes all my energy just to advocate for the care for my boys.

Tuesday, January 30, 2007
NICU Day 114

I t's been a long day with fussy babies. Fortunately for me, Nana comes by the hospital earlier than her usual time and holds the twins so I can run for a quick sandwich. The boys are cranky, but once in Nana's arms they fall fast asleep.

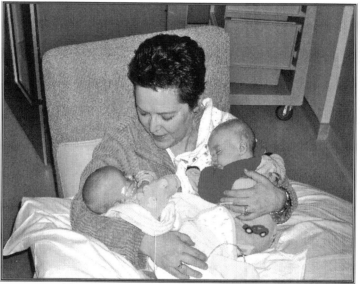

Nana calms two fussy babies - Ethan (left) and Aidan

As soon as Nana leaves for the day, both boys are howling again. To comfort the babies, I place Aidan in bed with Ethan, and Ethan stops crying immediately. Aidan wails on a bit longer until he realizes he is the only baby still crying. He stares intently at his brother; then closes his eyes and falls fast asleep.

I take this quiet moment to get another round of breast pumping done. Draping a privacy shawl over me, I hook up both breasts to the electric pump. It's a simple routine I have repeated every three hours around the clock without a hitch for the past three months—except today I hit a snag.

Just as the pump cranks up, both babies wake and start to howl. What a sight. My boys are howling at the top of their lungs and I'm hooked to the electric breast pump. There is no nurse in sight to help. Frantic to calm the babies, I try singing a lullaby song—only this makes them cry louder.

Dr. Placket walks by the open door and with a brief glance he is able to assess the full situation. Breaking into a broad grin he sums up my entire future in ten words— "You'll definitely need help when you get both babies home!"

Saturday, February 3, 2007
NICU Day 118

No sense in posting to the journal every day; the days are all the same. Ethan is not moving dramatically ahead, nor is he falling behind—he just hovers in the middle.

Today is the day the boys would have been born if I had carried them to the full 40 weeks gestation. This means that while they are nearly four months old chronologically, their adjusted age is one day old.

***

We're moving at the pace Ethan sets. When he tires on the cannula after two hours, he's put back on CPAP to give his lungs a rest.

His stats took another dip today—the lungs are filling with fluid once again. The lower dose of prednisone is not working. The doctors step up steroids from 1.25 mg to 3.0 mg per day. Heavy doses of steroids can't be maintained forever and the doctors warn us this rollercoaster of up and down has to stop soon. If the steroids don't work, we will need to make the trach decision.

The afternoon stats actually improve a bit. Ethan's FiO_2 support was around 30-35% several days ago, and today it is down to 28-30%. The goal is to get this support down to 25%—darn close to room air of 21% oxygen. The doctors say they will watch Ethan's progress for one more week. If he is not close to coming off CPAP, they will talk about making plans for a tracheostomy.

I have a sense of foreboding. I am convinced trach surgery would be the beginning of the end for Ethan. These thoughts of doubt are tucked away in my journal. I just hope we won't have to face this dragon.

Sunday, February 4, 2007
NICU Day 119

D

r. Lesotho is planning extended time off and stops in to say goodbye. I wish him well. We've been together for so long and through so much; it seems like one of our family is leaving. We didn't always agree—but I know he cared passionately.

***

Dr. Placket brings up the trach discussion once again. "Around 80% of babies with health issues like Ethan's need a tracheostomy."

He clarifies this a bit adding that while most babies in this situation need a trach; it is a lower probability for Ethan—perhaps only a 60% chance because of Ethan's attitude. He describes this as Ethan's spunky approach to life.

He amplifies this gentle warning with a grim face.

"I am concerned Ethan might be faced with a lifetime of lung issues if we don't get this under control now."

To make sure I understand, he drives home the severity saying, "Ethan's lungs are so poor, if these lungs were in a 10 year old child he would not survive."

Tuesday, February 6, 2007
NICU Day 121

D r. Placket says he'll give Ethan another two weeks on prednisone, and then he will try to wean him from CPAP to the nasal cannula. So the trach decision is delayed for now. We are given two weeks breathing room; pardon the pun—and I feel pressure to meet this goal.

The trach decision has been pushed out several times already. Each time we get close to a deadline, Ethan seems to be on the brink of meeting the goal. The doctors want him to have every chance to make the transition off oxygen support without trach surgery.

The trick is not waiting too long to decide. If we wait too long, the risk is we could miss the opportune time before Ethan's health turns south again. If he has another infection or further failure with his lungs, Ethan could become too weak to survive surgery.

Dr. Placket is frank. "The continued lack of sustained progress is concerning. I scheduled the full team to convene for a Care Plan Consult. This is where the entire medical team meets with the family to discuss Ethan's prognosis and treatment strategy. The team will lay out the issues and the possible long-term implications."

The trach decision hangs in the air. But I know we can't continue in limbo.

Sunday, February 11, 2007
NICU Day 126

Today is Picture Day! I need something that feels normal—so I recruit Nurses Julie and Joan to help me take a family photo.

This is a comedy act. Nurse Julie has the camera; Justin holds Aidan; I hold Ethan; and Nurse Joan has the oxygen mask held up to Ethan's face.

When Julie says "Now" that is the clue for Joan to pull the mask away from Ethan's face and squat down quickly to get out of the picture. Over and over—place the mask on Ethan; give him a whiff of oxygen; squat down; CLICK!

This was organized chaos to get a photo. All of us are in tears from laughing. With all the commotion I was surprised Aidan slept through the whole affair. Ethan was so thrilled to be out of his plastic box he never took his eyes off of me.

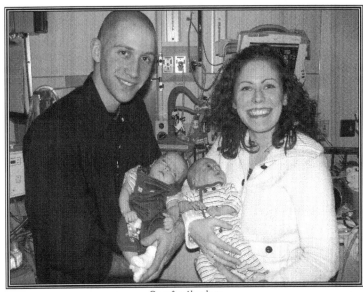

Our family photo

Monday, February 12, 2007
NICU Day 127

E than's hernias are much bigger. The stress of breathing with compromised lungs puts pressure on the lower intestines. This pressure causes his intestines to bulge out into his testicles through a hole created by the hernia—and they balloon up to the size of a small lemon.

The nurses show me how to manually press the intestines back into place. As long as there is no redness, and they slide back easily, we're okay.

Nana and I reduce the hernia with each diaper change, but Papa and Justin aren't too keen on doing this.

***

Ethan has a lot of progress to make before the upcoming Care Plan Consult. It's just 10 days away. In advance of this meeting, we hear pep talks from doctors, respiratory therapists, and nurses on the likelihood Ethan will need a trach. Their words are preparing us for the inevitable.

I am so tired.

I think Ethan is tired too.

If a trach is the only way for Ethan to recover, then I must agree.

Valentine's Day, Wednesday, February 14, 2007
NICU Day 129

E than has a special test today to see if he can handle the cannula for four hours straight *and* handle two feeding sessions by bottle. This is an important test, as it will help determine the answer to the trach question coming up.

The results are in—Ethan did well on this test!

Before I can get too jubilant, Dr. Lim issues a caution saying, "Passing one test does not mean anything concrete—just as failing one test does not set anything as final."

***

Reflux, reflux, reflux...Aidan continues to throw up everywhere. All my clothes are stained. The sofa is stained. Even the dog has baby vomit on him. I don't remember when I grocery shopped last. I hope Justin is feeding the pets, as I haven't in weeks. The last time I took a shower I closed my eyes and let the warm water pour over me. This way I get a three-minute nap and a shower at the same time.

Wednesday, February 21, 2007
NICU Day 136

My boss calls. There is an exciting new project at work and he wants to know if I can come back earlier than planned. My leave of absence is up on April 16, however he wants to know if I'd consider coming back this Monday. It is so tempting to think about re-entering the work world. I fantasize that I answer *Yes!*

Of course, that's not reality. I shake the fantasy dialogue from my head and tell him, "Thanks for the offer, but I think it will be best to wait until the April date."

To fill in the awkward silence that follows, I add; "We're going broke on one paycheck, so it is tempting; but I still have one baby in the hospital and I need this extra time to get my household in order."

I sense this was not the right response. My boss hems and haws a bit—then his voice becomes terse as he explains how hard this is on him.

There is no sense in laying out details as to why I can't return early. I don't think I could adequately explain this medical drama so anyone outside of the NICU world could understand what we're dealing with.

There are a lot of loose ends to resolve before my leave of absence is up. I haven't even figured out daycare yet. All my mental and emotional energies are consumed just handling day-to-day issues.

I offer to give my cell number to the temp employee who was hired to cover my desk while I'm on family-leave. Fortunately my boss does not take me up on this offer.

This phone call has me worried.

Once again I am reminded that my job is in jeopardy.

Chapter 25 - *Care Plan Consult*

*"What seems to us as bitter trials
are often blessings in disguise."*

Oscar Wilde

Thursday, February 22, 2007
NICU Day 137

Today is the much anticipated consult meeting. The whole medical team is here. Several even come in on their day off. Justin, however, is presenting a bid that is a make-it or break-it deal for his company—so he's running late. If he doesn't land this contract, his company will not have enough revenue to continue.

Nana and Papa are here to lend support. Nana takes copious notes on the discussion so can I focus carefully to everything that is said.

Dr. Lim and Dr. Placket open the session by summing up the medical situation.

Lungs

"These lungs," says Dr. Placket, "are as bad as I have ever seen."

"X-rays show clinically Ethan should not be able to survive. But he is, and that's typical of Ethan's entire heath history which defies standard medical statistics."

Looking serious, he adds; "We'll hold off discussion on the trach until the end of this Care Consult."

Social Growth

Dr. Lim covers the next topic. "As a micro-preemie Ethan is quite advanced with his social interactions. We have to take into consideration social vulnerabilities of a micro-preemie to bond with his family. This is something I have no concerns with. In fact, I credit the tremendous social skills of Ethan—his eye contact and how he engages and interacts with his caregivers—as no accident. I attribute this to Jen's mothering skills and the attention he is given from the rest of his family, including Aidan."

Okay, I feel suitably flattered at this.

He nods in Papa and Nana's direction, saying, "The family's constant presence at the hospital has been a significant factor in Ethan's progress. In fact, I would say Ethan's social interactions greatly influenced my decisions on pushing the envelope and advocating for Ethan well beyond what common practice might say is standard."

Growth and Nutrition

The nutritionist is up next and she says; "Ethan's extremely low birth weight made it difficult for me to gauge the proper blend of calories and additives. Ethan is such a tiny baby that even 137 days post birth, he is only just now big enough to plot on a preemie growth chart."

"The extremely low birth weight means Ethan will have a difficult time growing and developing normally. Bones need calcium and phosphorus—but we had to constantly back off these fortifiers while Ethan was on steroids. This is one of the reasons why he has rickets and will be prone to developing arthritis later in life.

"Ethan will continue to have growth issues—and I am concerned he could be a *failure to thrive*[25] baby. This will need very close monitoring."

Motor Skills

The physical therapist notes, "Ethan's muscle tone is affected by his emotional state. When he is calm and not stressed, he can keep his head straight. However, when he is tired or agitated he cannot hold his head up. Ethan is at

---

[25] *Failure to thrive* lacks a precise definition, in part because it describes a condition rather than a specific disease. Kids who fail to thrive are unable to take in, retain, or utilize the calories needed to gain weight and grow. Most diagnoses of failure to thrive are made in infants and toddlers in the first few years of life—a crucial period of physical and mental development. After birth, a child's brain grows as much in the first year as it will grow during the rest of life. Poor nutrition during this period can have permanent negative effects on mental development.

great risk for problems with motor skills. If I had just seen Ethan on one of his bad days, I'd say he has cerebral palsy. But, I have also seen him on a calm day, and I am not so certain."

Parenting at Home

The nurses take turns giving their feedback. "Ethan will do fine at home. We've watched Jen and know she is able to interpret Ethan's signals and can anticipate his needs."

I did not realize so much of the Care Consult was about whether I could care for Ethan at home. They have been *watching me* as much as I have been *watching them!*

Cardiac

Dr. Placket explains, "Right now there are no signs of heart issues, but the extended doses of steroids combined with chronic lung disease can be problematic. They can cause an enlarged heart and other cardiac issues. Post-discharge Ethan will need to be assigned to a cardiologist for continued monitoring."

Vision and Hearing

"Ethan lost his peripheral vision due to ROP," says Dr. Lim. "Since he never had this range of vision, he won't realize it's gone. I suspect he may have issues with depth perception, and of course he'll need glasses."

"Also, heavy antibiotic use can cause severe loss of hearing. He may need a hearing specialist after discharge."

***

This is a long meeting, but no one is rushing to get through. Dr. Lim moves to a list of what happens when Ethan is ready to go home.

Oxygen

"Ethan will not be able to come off oxygen support until after he is successfully weaned off prednisone. He can go home with a portable oxygen tank when he's able to handle a low flow rate of 0.5 liters on the cannula."

Prednisone and Diuretics

"Ethan will need to continue on steroids even after he goes home to help his lungs recover. Unfortunately this can stunt growth and the side effects of long-term steroid use can lead to an enlarged heart, kidney failure, and brain issues including loss of motor skills. These issues will need constant monitoring by your pediatrician."

Trach or Cannula?

I expected to hear the final decision on trach surgery today, however Dr. Lim says; "I'm still not ready to say one way or the other on this matter. I did not bring the pulmonologist in for this consult meeting because I already know what he'd say. He would say a trach is definitely needed and that I should have ordered one some time ago."

Dr. Lim pauses, and then covers the points once again. "The pulmonologist would come to the correct decision based on stats, that surgery is needed. On the other hand, the doctors here know Ethan. We see him and we see the full picture of the family supporting Ethan. This baby has not followed a textbook course; therefore we've been more willing to wait a bit longer before making a big decision like this."

Putting on his stern face Dr. Lim adds; "If Ethan does not meet specific goals over the next two weeks, this will be out of my hands. I will be forced to go the trach route. Ethan's lungs are the worst I have ever seen in a surviving preemie. If we can't reach the oxygen goals, I will be forced to order a trach."

No one says anything for the longest time. It is in this moment of silence I see more fully the battle Dr. Lim has been fighting.

He has been under considerable pressure to make a decision in favor of the trach. Dr. Lim has fought back against this pressure—but he will cede the point if Ethan can't maintain his oxygen levels.

Post-Discharge Medical Team

The consult meeting ends with a list of post discharge responsibilities. No date is selected yet, but we are told of the number of doctors that we will need to line up to care for Ethan after his discharge. He will need a primary care pediatrician with a specialty in high-risk babies as well as a suite of specialists including: pulmonologist; neurologist; cardiologist; surgeon for hernia repair; gastroenterologist; ophthalmologist; and a full set of physical, speech, and nutrition therapists.

Talk about your million-dollar baby. I wonder how all these specialists will be paid once Ethan leaves the hospital.

Sunday, February 25, 2007
NICU Day 140

The hearing test is today. I'm a bit anxious, as the doctors have repeatedly warned Ethan has an increased probability of being a deaf child. Prolonged doses of potent antibiotics and steroids can cause severe hearing loss. This possibility has been nagging in the back of my mind for some time now.

My university studies were in the field of Special Ed with a major in Deaf Education. Before making the big change in direction of my career into financial services, I worked with special needs kids. This included work with deaf children and those with autism, Down's syndrome, cerebral palsy, and vision impairments. I know some of the challenges a family faces with a special needs child.

The hearing test is over and the doctor comes to our NICU room to tell me the results.

He is smiling from ear to ear.

My eyes tear up in relief with his unspoken good news.

Tuesday, February 27, 2007
NICU Day 142

I t's a bad day today. Ethan has labored breathing. Each breath rattles with a pronounced wet and raspy sound. I feel this is an ominous sign. Even the body language of the nursing staff and respiratory therapists show they too feel defeated.

Thursday, March 1, 2007
NICU Day 144

D r. Baillie pops in to see us during rounds. He's a distinguished looking doctor—so it is a bit incongruous to see him literally bouncing on his toes bursting with good news.

"It may be possible for Ethan to be at home on a higher flow cannula!" he says. "There's a new machine available for home use." The words hardly leave his mouth when he hurries off to discuss this idea with Dr. Lim.

Of course I stopped hearing anything after the words *"...Ethan at home..."* I savor them. Is Ethan really turning the corner? Why, it was just the other day my baby had such labored breathing even the nurses looked depressed.

***

Our pediatrician is making plans for taking on Ethan's care after our son is discharged from the NICU. The doctor calls me to go over the details.

"I consider Ethan to be a *red card* baby," he says.

Dr. Clausen explains this means our appointments are top priority and we will get the coveted early morning time slot. Also, we will avoid the waiting room full of sick kids, as we are to bring Ethan through a private back door and head directly to the exam room.

I chuckle to myself at the words *red card*. Ethan hasn't played his first soccer game and he is already 'red carded'!

My mind briefly wanders as I imagine Ethan and Aidan running across the soccer fields dressed in matching uniforms—with their little legs pumping hard as they run to kick the ball.

This is the first time I have daydreamed about my children's future since they were born.

Friday, March 2, 2007
NICU Day 145

Ethan's breathing is not as labored today. My spirits are up after several days of worry that he might not make the transition to the cannula. I think he may have found the road home at last. My personal goal is to have Ethan home by the 16th of March—my 30th birthday. All I want for my birthday is both of my sons at home.

***

Just when I relax, another setback occurs. After I leave the NICU for the day, a new rotation doctor puts Ethan on a changed feeding schedule. She orders the nurse to give Ethan as much formula as he wants, when he wants it. The unfortunate timing of assigning a new doctor is this occurs on the same day Ethan is has a new nightshift nurse. Now Ethan has two new people who are not aware of his tendency to have trouble handling changes in feeding routines.

Ethan gorges himself on this new schedule and throws up all his feeds and meds several times. This upsets him, which in turn distresses his breathing and puts a strain on his lungs.

Damn it! This order to change feedings never should have been made. Perhaps the new doctor misread Ethan's happy demeanor as a sign that she could push him to the next level of treatment. After he threw up the first time, Ethan should have put back on scheduled feeds. Unfortunately, the changed schedule was left in place, so Ethan repeated this cycle of gorging and vomiting again and again all night long.

Weeks of progress have been dashed by one foolish change in a feeding schedule.

Saturday, March 3, 2007
NICU Day 146

E than is still agitated this morning after last night's feeding disaster. Nurse Julie sees right away what the problem is and talks with Dr. Baillie. He agrees Ethan needs to go back to the three-hour feeding cycle.

I am so upset, but as the morning wears on and Ethan bounces back, I realize I am making far too much of this. Babies throw up, plain and simple. This is not a federal case and certainly not worth all the drama I wrapped around it in my journal posting.

I have not slept through a single night in 146 days.

Sleep deprivation and post-partum depression—what a combination.

I have got to get some sleep.

Monday, March 5, 2007
NICU Day 148

D
r. Lim and Dr. Placket have big smiles today. They say we can start thinking about bringing Ethan home. I'm in hyper-drive to get everything ready as I check off my massive to-do list.

Oxygen
A supply of oxygen tanks is delivered to our home. These come in several sizes. The 5-foot tall tank is placed in the upstairs nursery. It looks like a big torpedo. There is a mid-size tank in the family room and a small portable one is stashed in the car for trips to the doctor's office. A week's supply of spare tanks in all sizes fills our garage.

The local fire station is notified about the oxygen stored in the house and about Ethan's medical situation in case we have to call 911.

Monitors
We are shown how to place the oximeter monitor on Ethan's foot to check his blood oxygen levels. Dr. Placket quizzes us on what steps to take when the alarm sounds— what vitals to monitor first, when to trigger CPR, and when to call 911.

CPR
Justin, Nana, Papa and I took a CPR course when Aidan was discharged—and now we take a refresher class. We pay close attention and practice on the infant-sized dummy. You never saw such serious students. We know our stuff.

Feeding Tube
I am shown how to insert the feeding tube down Ethan's nose and how to check to be sure it ended up with

the correct placement in his stomach. The nurses tell me they don't normally send a baby home with a feeding tube, but Ethan is a special case and they trust me to do it correctly. I feel in the last five months I've become an honorary nurse.

Medications and Feedings

The doctors go over the long list of medications and the instructions on how to mix the complicated prescription formula. I think my kitchen will be turned into a pharmacy.

Car Seat

Ethan passes the car seat test. This means while wearing a cannula for oxygen support, he can sit upright for 30 minutes without a major breathing issue.

My eyes follow the length of the cannula tubing as it snakes to the oxygen tank. This tank will somehow need to be wedged in next to Ethan' car seat. I make a mental note to ask Justin to rig up some sort of safety strap so it doesn't turn into a flying missile in a sudden stop.

Follow-Up Appointments

There will be almost daily appointments after we leave the hospital. The doctors say this is a borderline decision to discharge Ethan—but I am sure I can take care of my babies at home.

I briefly wonder how I will handle getting the twins to all their doctor appointments after I return to work.

No room for doubts now.

Chapter 26 - *Ethan's Day*

"Hope is like a road in the country;
there was never a road,
but when many people walk on it,
the road comes into existence."

Lin Yutang

Ethan's Day - Friday, March 9, 2007
NICU Day 152

Today Ethan is coming home. A date we will celebrate each year as 'Ethan's Day'. Born five months ago with an APGAR score of 2 and weighing not much more than a pound, my son is finally able to leave the hospital weighing in at whooping 8 lbs. 15 oz. (4064 grams).

It is bittersweet leaving the hospital today. We've come to regard the whole medical team as family.

There are many tears of happiness as Ethan is wished farewell. I am already looking forward to a five-year reunion visit with our NICU family when I plan to bring the boys back to show off our sons all grown up.

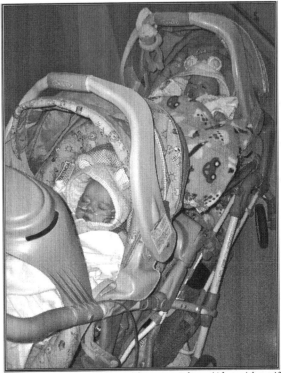

Leaving the NICU – Ethan with oxygen tubes; Aidan with pacifier

The doctors warn me it is likely Ethan's health will fail again and he will need to be brought back to the hospital— as almost all micro-preemies have repeat hospitalizations.

I hear this warning and intentionally downplay the meaning. Right now my mind is overwhelmed as I mentally sort and re-organize every little detail of how to handle two fragile babies at home.

***

I view this as the next chapter of our lives where our babies are to grow healthier every day.

Five months ago I desperately wanted to know, *did anyone ever make it out of the NICU?* I needed to know that a baby could survive against the toughest odds.

During the past five months, hope was often allusive and so hard to see. And yet it was always there, just waiting for me to find it.

Many babies traveled this path before us; some made it home and some did not. Each one showed the medical community a way to help future preemies survive. I thank these babies for showing the way. And I am forever grateful to all families that traveled this road ahead of us.

Tuesday, March 13, 2007
Age 5 months 4 days

With two babies at home, there is no sleeping in this house, not even for the dog. Poor Jameson is sprayed with baby vomit when he comes too close investigating the second boy taking up residence in his house. I'll bathe the dog tomorrow. Our first days at home are too chaotic.

How will I handle two babies around the clock?

I am fixated on the topic of sleep—I know now why *sleep deprivation* is considered a method of torture!

Do they have a Geneva Convention for new moms?

***

I have a spiral notepad I affectionately call the "In and Out" book. Here is where anyone helping me with the babies enters notes on feedings, vomit, pee and bowel movements. We also record times for medications, blood oxygen oximeter readings, and questions I need to remember to ask the pediatrician. It is too hard for me to keep track of which baby did what by memory, so I rely on the "In and Out" log to keep a sense of order in this chaos.

I am happy and—even though I am in a perpetual fog of exhaustion—I have a silly grin on my face as I stare at my miracle babies.

Life is far from normal. The boys don't seem to sleep at the same time. One of the twins is always in the midst of eating, vomiting, or crying. When they do finally fall asleep, I grab the camera and take their precious picture.

Everywhere Ethan goes he is tethered to an oxygen tank. I can't freely move him from room-to-room, as there's a limit to the length of the oxygen tubing.

Ethan has patches of Velcro tape on his cheeks—these hold the oxygen tubing in place. The tape is tough on his skin and I've been warned about potential for facial scars if this adhesive is left in place too long. Extra care is taken to gently soak the tape off and move it to a new spot on his face every few days.

The regiment of medications is overwhelming. Ethan has to take a constant dose of diuretics and steroids to pull fluid out of his lungs. The trouble is the taste. Nana tested a miniscule amount on tip of her tongue and she reports they taste horrendous!

It literally takes me a full 60 minutes to get Ethan to eat his cocktail of formula spiked with meds. In less than ten seconds he throws everything back up. We lose the medication and all the precious food that took forever to get down this baby.

At first I fed Ethan through the NG tube. However, after three days at home, he figured out how to pull out all 25 centimeters of the tubing and left it for me to find in his crib. Now that he knows this trick, he pulls the tubing out immediately after I get it re-inserted.

I can't get the tube into his nose and down his throat any more. Ethan screams and looks at me like I'm torturing him. His throat is so raw and swollen. Guess we will have to manage by just using a bottle—I can't force this anymore.

***

I stop by the pharmacy to pick up Ethan's prescription formula. Like Aidan's formula, this too is a special high-calorie blend only available by prescription. The pharmacist says this is a custom order—and I have to pay for it in advance because our medical insurance plan *specifically excludes* prescription formula.

He wants $900 payment up front to fill a one-month supply for two babies. I am in tears. How can I pay for this? We've asked for financial help and we're told we do not qualify because we have health insurance.

The pharmacist with an air of confidentiality stage-whispers to me; "If you just cancel your health insurance, these prescriptions would be paid for by Medicaid."

Is that what it takes to get help? What's wrong with this system?

I leave the pharmacy empty handed.

Fortunately my pediatrician gave me a small supply of samples from his office. This will last for a few days while I figure out a way to leverage one more credit card to pay for a monthly supply of formula.

Friday, March 16, 2007
Age 5 months 7 days

Today is my 30ᵗʰ birthday. I got what I wanted—both boys home from the hospital. Justin asks what I want for my birthday gift. The answer I give is simple; "I want to sleep."

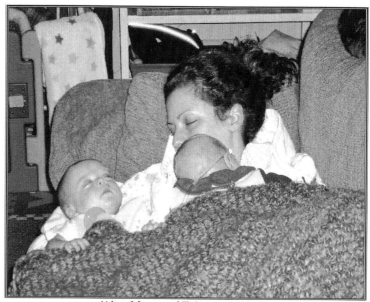

Aidan, Mama and Ethan - asleep at last

We celebrate my birthday with a short party at Nana and Papa's house. I receive a gift certificate for the beauty salon. Seems a lifetime ago since I had my hair or nails done!

After the celebratory dinner, it's time to pack up the babies and head home to start the cycle of feeding, vomiting, and changing oxygen tanks all over again.

The last five months have been spent in survival mode. Justin and I did what was needed to get by. Our marriage didn't fall apart, but it wasn't exactly the ideal marriage either. We both focused on what we had to do to survive this hell—me tending to the boys and Justin working two jobs.

Once the twins were home from the hospital, I thought this survival mode would be over. How disappointing to find this is not the case. Leaving the hospital didn't make things better. I still struggle every minute of every day with the health of my children.

I can't do anything other than care for them, and most of the time I'm not enough. Help is needed with even the most basic task, like feeding both babies. It takes over an hour to get Ethan to take his formula spiked with meds. Aidan can't be left unattended for an hour, so in each three-hour window of time, I need at least one hour of help.

I'm overwhelmed.

The light I expected to find once the boys were discharged from the hospital isn't there after all.

Chapter 27 - *Reflux Reflux Reflux*

"Are we not like two volumes of one book?"

Marceline Desbordes-Valmor

Monday, March 19, 2007
Age 5 months 10 days

Both boys have reflux. At least when Aidan spits up, he is willing to replace the lost food with another bottle. Ethan on the other hand, falls into a very deep sleep and won't wake up for any more feedings. The strain of eating is too much—he has no energy to do anything except breathe.

To help out, my family fills in where they can. Nana helps during the hectic early evening hours after she leaves her office. For the long daytime hours, Papa is here to help me with babies, pets, and house chores. Our wonderful friends and neighbors bring over meals. I couldn't make it if not for this support.

I was able to leave the house for an hour today to use my gift certificate at the beauty salon. Justin stayed home with the boys. I'm not sure who ended up in charge, but Justin sure needed a beer when I got back.

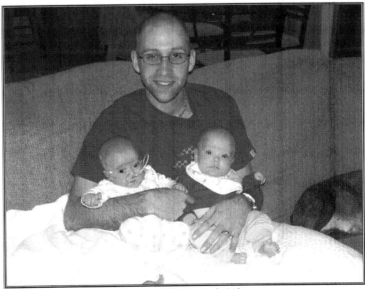

Justin with Ethan and Aidan

Tuesday, March 20, 2007
Age 5 months 11 days

I am getting close to the end of my leave of absence from work. Our original plan was to place the babies in the daycare facility located across the street from my office building. The doctor says Ethan's lungs are too fragile to be exposed to daycare—so I will have to hire someone for in-home care instead.

Researching nanny care is underway in earnest. I briefly considered using a placement company that lines up students from abroad to work as a live-in nanny. But we don't have a spare bedroom; and besides, I need someone with experience to handle medically fragile babies.

The cost is distressing. In-home care cost more than daycare—in fact, a nanny will cost more than my net take-home salary. So in effect, I will be working just for benefits.

My return to work date is April 16—less than a month away. I don't know how I'm going to handle this. Even with a nanny, I still have to get the boys to their doctor visits. With two babies averaging three specialist's appointments each week, I'll be leaving work early nearly every day. How can I work and cover all these doctor appointments?

***

While we try to figure out my work situation, Justin is forced to give up his dream of building his own company. He tells his business partner they are out of revenue. Justin will have to close up his firm and find some kind of corporate job that will offer us a fixed income and a health insurance plan.

It is such a shame to lose the company he built.

We are exhausted and out of options.

I can't believe we have money worries on top of everything else. We waited and built a strong financial base before starting our family. We both had good jobs. We had health insurance. We saved and bought a house with a fixed-rate mortgage. Our credit score was stellar and we had no credit card debt. Stashed in the bank was enough savings to last for a year and our two IRA accounts were accumulating a nice cushion for our future.

I feel naïve. If we had been without health insurance, Medicaid would have covered our medical bills; but because we have insurance and are employed, we're not eligible for help. I thought we were financially smart, but it looks like we're going to lose every last dime.

I feel betrayed. My employer (a $28 billion asset financial services company) selected a health plan for its employees with more holes in it than a sieve. This insurance—for which I pay a hefty monthly premium—provides no more protection than a house of cards. This policy had dumped us into a hole of medical bills so deep we'll never be able to climb out.

Thursday, March 22, 2007
Age 5 months 13 days

Today is a weight check at the pediatrician's. It's a challenge to get both boys bundled up and out of the house on any sort of time schedule. I feel like a pack-mule as I firmly grasp the handles of two car seats with the babies strapped inside. A diaper bag of supplies is slung on one shoulder and a portable oxygen tank lies strapped across my back.

I am learning where to find parking spots with access ramps for the double stroller and stalls wide enough so I can open the car doors fully to remove each infant seat.

The rare parking spots that can accommodate us are a long walk from the doctor's office. There are reserved spots for disabled parking—why can't there be parking stalls reserved for parents with strollers?

Unloading the car is a circus act. First I lug the double-long stroller out of the trunk and set the brake so it won't roll away. I cram Ethan's oxygen tank into the bottom of the stroller—it looks like a torpedo sticking out the back end. Next, I snap each car seat into place on the stroller and reconnect Ethan to his oxygen tank. The diaper bag hangs off the stroller handle and I stuff my wallet and car keys into the side pocket. Blankets and baby hats (it's cold here in March) are firmly tucked in place.

Now I have to get from the parking garage; across the outdoor lot; into the medical building; up the elevator; and into the doctor's office before one of the babies starts crying. If they cry, they vomit, and if they vomit, you better not be leaning over them saying, 'Oh my, what a cute baby'. The projectile vomit will fill your face and run down your collar. Ask me how I know.

Monday, April 2, 2007
Age 5 months 24 days

Carting a tiny baby tethered to an oxygen tank takes extra planning. Even in the house I can't move from room to room without wheeling an oxygen tank along. It has become second nature now.

When an empty tank needs to be swapped out, I can slap the nozzles together in just seconds—almost as fast as Justin.

A device to monitor blood oxygen saturation is placed on Ethan's foot and held in place with special non-stick tape and covered with a bootie. At night the game is to see how long the monitor will stay on before our little Houdini Escape Artist is able to kick it off. Ethan's record is less than one minute. Each time the monitor is kicked off, the alarm sounds and I have to go check on him. When I enter the nursery, Ethan greets me with a wide smile—as if to say, "Hi Mama! Isn't this a fun game?"

Bath time is comical. I fill the tub with an inch of water and make sure the room is toasty warm. Aidan lies naked on the bath carpet waiting his turn while I bathe Ethan. The oxygen tank is propped next to the tub and I try to keep the cannula tubes from falling into the water. The dog loves bath time and he thinks the water is just for him. I use a body-block move to keep Jameson from jumping into the tub with Ethan and this makes me loosen my grip on the oxygen tubes. As the tubing falls into the water with a splash, Aidan has to pee and shoots urine all over me. Jameson heads out of the bathroom carrying off one of the dirty diapers. The phone is ringing, and the oxygen delivery guy is knocking at the front door.

They can all wait.

It's bath time.

This is my relaxing time of the day.

Thursday, April 12, 2007
Age 6 months 4 days

L uckily, Justin found a job as a project manager with a commercial flooring firm. He also takes on side-jobs to supplement our income. It is an 80-hour workweek for him, but at last we have a consistent salary flow.

Justin is excited with the opportunities with his new employer—however we have to wait three months for medical benefits to start. The hope is his insurance plan will cover the balances not paid for by my health plan. With two insurance policies we expect 100% coverage; or so we think. Unfortunately the additional medical plan has exclusions as well, so we are still exposed to significant balances.

I head back to work this coming Monday. It will be a relief to get the second salary started up again. Of course, I am fretting about having to leave the babies with someone else.

We found a nanny—an older woman from the neighborhood. Her salary will take up nearly all of my paycheck. Once the boys grow stronger and healthy enough to handle a public setting, we will switch to the less costly alternative of daycare. We just have to find a way for our finances to last until then.

A fast tour through the closet and I have my office clothes laid out. What a relief—they still fit.

I just finish typing the daily schedule of medications and feeding instructions for the nanny when the phone rings. Caller ID shows it's her calling. I figure she wants to go over some last minute details.

Her words shock me.

"I have been having second thoughts," she says. "Taking care of babies on oxygen tanks and all their complicated formulas and medications…well Honey…this is just too much. I am so sorry."

She quit before she even started!

What am I going to do? Shall I just tuck the babies in my briefcase and take them to work with me on Monday? I would have liked more notice—but I did suspect anyone we hired would quit eventually, as they would tire of the constant care my boys require.

I am resigned to the situation. This means I can't go back to work and I know we're in a financial free-fall.

This bad news can wait—I'll tell Justin after he gets home tonight.

***

It is well past 9:30 PM before Justin finally makes it home. He put in long day at his new job and has the added stress of closing down his own company. And of course, he too gets no sleep.

Tonight of all nights I have no sympathy for his long day, as my husband forgot to stop by the pharmacy on his way home.

Justin says he'll go right back out. That doesn't cut it with me. I play the martyr as if forgetting to stop at the pharmacy is an unforgivable transgression that only I can make right.

"The boys are out of their meds. *I will go myself.*"

The truth is I want to get out of the house—even if it's just a 10-minute trip to the pharmacy.

What a sight I am—baby-puke covered sweat pants and disheveled hair. The cashier commiserates with me saying her kids were practically twins as they were only 10 months apart—so she knows exactly what I am going through.

I think to myself, *oh no you don't!*

The cashier chides me for not clipping the coupon from today's paper. She digs through the check-stand drawers to find a one-dollar discount coupon for pharmacy refills.

I don't mind that she's holding up the line. I use this delay as a way to steal 40-winks.

My out-of-pocket cost for the refill prescriptions this week is $197.40. I slap down a credit card praying there is enough credit balance left to cover this charge.

Friday, April 13, 2007
Age 6 months 5 days

It's Friday the 13th. How appropriate. I call work and let them know our childcare plan didn't work out. I can't return to work on Monday after all. The conversation with my boss is brief. I'll call the HR office next and work out the details of my resignation. I should feel bad about giving them such short notice, but I am just numb.

I don't know what else to do. How will we survive this? With this one phone call I have just killed seven years worth of my career in the financial services industry.

Finishing these calls, I turn my attention back to Ethan. He's been quiet while I was on the phone. That's not normal. I should have a fussy baby.

Something is wrong!

Ethan is listless and spiking a high temperature.

I place a quick call to Nana and she leaves her office right away to come help. We can't get any fluids into Ethan with the bottle, so I use an eyedropper to dribble Pedialyte™ into his mouth. We are trying desperately to get fluid into this baby. He won't swallow and is so listless.

As the fever climbs above 104°F, I rush Ethan off to the hospital.

The emergency room doctor says this is pneumonia. The plan is to admit Ethan to the hospital and push IV fluids. I find some good news in all this mess—this is plain old pneumonia and not the dreaded RSV.

Ethan has thrown up all over me so many times tonight my sweater can stand up on its own. I look (and smell) frightful. I think I'm coming down with the flu bug too, as I feel a fever coming on.

Justin, Aidan, Nana, and Papa are all sick with the flu as well. I don't even want to think of what it is like at my house right now.

It wasn't supposed to be like this. Once discharged from the NICU we were supposed to be on the road to recovery. Sure, I knew it would be gradual, but I did not expect this many setbacks to plague us.

Since the boys were born we have been living a cycle of days and nights filled with fear, depression, frustration, sadness, guilt, disappointment, and self-doubt. Discharge from the NICU did not stop the roller coaster ride; it just made it lonelier.

I still feel as if I'm in survival mode. I don't feel like myself at all. I'm tired all the time. I'm scared of what's going to happen to us financially. I'm constantly worried about the boys' health. I miss my life. I'm putting every ounce of myself into being a good mom—and I know I'm not being a good wife.

Justin is holding our family together. I'm lucky he is such a patient man. Justin takes the burden of this catastrophic year in his own stoic way and patiently waits for me to come back to myself.

I just hope I can come back.

Wednesday, April 18, 2007
Age 6 months 10 days

It took three days for Ethan to recover enough lung power to be discharged from the hospital, however he still requires more oxygen flow than usual. Ethan's little chest heaves and nostrils flare as he sucks in air. My son has to fight to breathe, which makes him anxious and in turn causes more labored breathing.

I hook-up a blow-by—meaning I let a stream of oxygen blow across his nose. This rush of air calms Ethan and helps him remember to take deeper breaths. This also uses up oxygen at a faster rate than normal.

A call is placed to the oxygen supply company to have more tanks delivered. The guy on the phone gives me a really hard time about going through oxygen too quickly.

He says I should have ordered more tanks to begin with, as now he will be inconvenienced having to make a mid-week delivery.

I think to myself, *you're harassing me about this when I have a sick baby at home? I don't care about your stupid delivery schedule. Just deliver the damn tanks.*

Chapter 28 - *Feeding Tube*

"Hope perches in the soul,
and sings a tune without words
and never stops it's singing;
even though at times you do not hear it."

Emily Dickinson

Wednesday, April 25, 2007
Age 6 months 17 days

The twins' calendar fills with several specialist appointments every month. Today's office visit is with our wonderful pediatrician, Dr. Clausen.

He tells me, "Ethan's significant lack of weight gain means he will face lifelong health and developmental issues. We have to get on top of this. If Ethan does not gain weight soon, we will need to consider having a G-tube implanted in his belly."

What's a G-tube?

"Gastrostomy surgery is where a tube is inserted from outside the abdomen—about two inches above the belly button—into the stomach. The tube would be left in place for a year or so, or until he gains weight; whichever is longer. Ethan would take his feeds with a bottle, and when he is too tired he can get the balance of his feedings through the G-tube."

Dr. Clausen glances over at his desk calendar.

"I'd like you to book an appointment now with the surgeon. It will take some time to get onto the surgical schedule; perhaps by the July or August timeframe."

We had finally stopped worrying about the trach surgery and now they want to cut a hole in my baby's belly to insert a feeding tube.

Dr. Clausen tells me to wean Ethan down from his medications and oxygen before the gastrostomy surgery. Over the next month I am to give Ethan as much solid food as he tolerates. This is for oral stimulation so he won't develop a total aversion to eating once the G-tube is surgically implanted.

I laugh when the doctor tells me not to increase the volume of formula just yet.

Increase the volume? Heck, I can hardly get Ethan to take anything now—how could I possibly increase the volume?

Friday, May 11, 2007
Age 7 months 3 days

At seven months old the boys get their first outing (other than to the hospital or doctor's office). Nana and I pile them into the car and head to Babies-R-Us to stock up on supplies. People stare at us as we parade through the store with little Ethan hooked up to his tank of oxygen.

The boys are such good shoppers that we decide to push our luck and make a quick stop at the Starbucks next door before heading back across the parking lot to our car.

I get in line to place our order, while Nana navigates the double-long stroller to a quiet corner of the coffee shop. The boys are so tiny they're hard to see tucked deep inside their infant seats.

It's funny the questions I am asked. Like the lady in the coffee line who says, "Do you ever take them out by yourself?"

I feel like saying, "No, they sometimes go out by themselves."

Or the one who asks, "Do they cry at the same time?"

Of course not! My boys are so polite they *take turns* crying.

My all time favorite; "Do they sleep through the night?"

Now I ask you. Do I *look* like I have slept the night through in the past 213 days?

Both boys are teething, which makes for fussy days. Amazingly, they get the same two front teeth on the same day. Their smiles are priceless.

The twins are now 7½ months old. Aidan is 13 lb. 7 oz., but Ethan continues his struggle to gain weight. He burns so many calories just breathing he is not putting on weight as he should. Ethan weighs a whooping three pounds less than Aidan—and most the weight he does have is from fluid retention attributed to his steroid meds.

Oxygen therapy continues and Ethan is allowed an hour break twice a day—mostly unscheduled breaks, as he tends to pull the cannula out of his nostrils by himself. I'll glance over and see he has pulled the oxygen tube from his nose and has the little rubber prongs stuck in his mouth (or ear, chin, etc.). The little imp is so clever he can dismantle the oxygen tubing taped to his face in less than a minute. He does it all with such a big smile, it distracts you for a few moments before you realize what he's done.

At night I set up the video baby monitor in the boys' room. If I hear a noise, I look at the monitor screen on my bedside table before deciding if I need to jump out of bed.

Tonight I hear a new sound come over the monitor. It is not the beeping of the oximeter alarm; it is the sound of laughter!

The boys are lying side-by-side in the crib they share. As they lift their legs straight up, their little sleeping sacks pop up like tents. This makes them giggle and laugh.

The sound is so precious and the sight of them popping their legs up and down as they wave their sleeping gowns makes me laugh aloud. I give Justin a poke in the ribs to wake him so he too can watch on the monitor. We lie there and snuggle together watching our sons at play.

Friday, June 29, 2007
Age 8 months 23 days

We're at Mercy Hospital for an MRI scan to check the progress of Ethan's brain bleed. I take off his clothes and dress him in a miniature hospital gown. The gown looks just like an adult-size one, but it is so tiny it would fit a 14" baby doll.

I carry Ethan in my arms into the MRI room. He is happy and animated—until he sees doctors wearing scrubs and masks. Fast as lightening, he tries to climb up and over my shoulder as if to escape this place.

The nurse takes Ethan from me and lays him on the table. She gently, but firmly, pins the shoulders down as a doctor places the anesthesia mask over Ethan's face.

My baby's eyes dart around the room frantically searching for me. Ethan is crying silently into the facemask and asking me with his eyes to make this stop.

I smile and say reassuring words until he is sedated. Once Ethan is asleep, I crumple into tears and someone leads me out of the room.

Nana keeps me company as I pace the waiting room. She talks constantly; like a sideline coach trying to keep my spirits up.

When Ethan is wheeled back from the exam room my worries about him being back on the ventilator are unfounded. He came off the vent just fine and is breathing on his own with just supplemental oxygen.

The doctor tells me the scan shows no new problems with the brain bleeds. We're all so relieved.

I tuck the miniature gown into my diaper bag and pack up to leave the hospital. Maybe I will frame this gown and hang it next to Ethan's soccer jersey when he is a teenager.

Monday, July 2, 2007
Age 8 months 25 days

Less than a week later and we're back again to Mercy Hospital—this time for a heart scan. I try to keep Ethan entertained in the tiny consultation room while the cardiologist looks over the results on the computer monitor.

"With chronic lung disease the heart works harder to pump blood through the lungs," the doctor says waving his hand at the display image. "This impacts the heart muscles and can lead to enlargement of one of the chambers. Additionally, heart problems are linked to long-term use of antibiotics, steroids, and serotonin inhibitors such as dopamine."

The doctor turns his chair around to sit facing me.

I recognize this body language—he has bad news.

"While Ethan was in the NICU, it was anticipated he might develop heart issues. So it is not unexpected for me to find Ethan's aorta is distended. This is called aortic root dilatation. This has to do with where the ascending aorta connects to the heart. When the diameter of the aorta is too large, it causes blood to backwash in the reverse direction as the heart is pumping. In some cases this enlarged area can weaken and rupture."

Rupture? I am desperate to hear him say this will turn out okay.

"There is not much we can do now. We'll monitor this carefully over the next few years, and if the diameter continues to expand, there are treatments—such as medication to control blood pressure or heart surgery."

"Can this rupture if he's active or stressed?" I ask.

"No, not as a toddler—this is a concern in older kids. We'll have lots of warnings—so not to worry right now."

I tuck the information in the back of my brain and know we'll just have to add this to the list of things to monitor as Ethan grows up.

Monday, July 16, 2007
Age 9 months 9 days

We meet today with the surgeon who will perform Ethan's gastrostomy surgery. I don't recall his name—just that he has bright red curly hair. Shows you how pre-occupied I was throughout this meeting. I can't even hold on to simple things like people's names.

The doctor explains the G-tube surgery. He'll cut an incision into the stomach and insert a plug that will hook up to a feeding tube.

The doctor shows us how to assemble the feeding equipment. He shares photographs of babies where the surgery worked well—and pictures where the surgical site eroded away because of infection or because the tube was dislodged. The photos are disturbingly graphic.

My mind is reeling. How will we ever manage this? How will Ethan handle this? Can we keep the tube in place without him pulling it out? After all, this is the Houdini Escape Artist who ripped out IVs and tugged at oxygen masks in the NICU.

I have a bad feeling Ethan will not react well to this invasion of his body. Even so, I agree and the surgery date is set for August 29th—a little over a month from now.

They will do the hernia surgery at the same time and we'll finally get these herniated intestines held securely in their rightful place.

Wednesday, August 29, 2007
Age 10 months 23 days

Today is Ethan's hernia surgery. The original plan was to do the G-tube surgery today as well—but Ethan threw a delightful wrench into this plan. Surprise! Over the past month he has been gaining weight. The pediatrician joked with me the last time we were in for a weight check, asking if I put rocks in Ethan's socks!

While Ethan is only 12½ pounds—rather small for a nine-month-old baby—the weight gain is moving in the right direction at last.

The G-tube surgery is temporarily postponed. If he keeps gaining weight, this particular surgery will be cancelled altogether. If not, we will be back on the surgery schedule to slap a G-tube in this kid's belly.

Chapter 29 - *No More Oxygen!*

*"What oxygen is to the lungs,
such is hope to the meaning of life."*

Emil Brunner

Monday, September 10, 2007
Age 11 months 1 day

Aidan is crawling everywhere and Ethan seems envious. He watches Aidan and wants to be mobile as well. Ethan can get up on all fours and manages a rocking motion, but hasn't quite figured out how to put it all together to propel him forward. Even if he did figure this out he couldn't get far; the oxygen tubes tangle around his legs and tether him in place.

I don't know how I'm going to keep them corralled when they're both on the move. This all seems pretty remarkable; not so long ago we faced the prediction of a high chance of disabling cerebral palsy.

***

Much to my surprise at today's check-up, Dr. Clausen says Ethan can come off all oxygen support! Nearly a year old and this boy breathes for the first time in his life without the help of an oxygen tank.

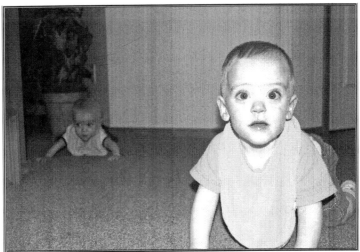

Aidan showing Ethan how to put crawling motions together

***

At this afternoon's physical therapy session, the therapist tries to engage Aidan in play-tasks. She notes he is uncooperative and will not make eye contact. This might be a sign of social interaction problems, such as Sensory Integration Disorder (SID). It is too early to tell if Aidan suffers from this—she just wants me to know what signs to watch for.

The physical therapist explains that preemies are at a high risk for autism and SID. Toddlers with SID perceive information differently than most people, as they have difficulty taking in, processing, and responding to stimulus. The signs to look for are extreme avoidance of certain activities, unexplained agitation, distress, fear, or confusion. These children will often clamp their hands over their eyes or ears to block stimulus.

I make a mental note to post this information to my journal when we get home. I have my hands too full right now to take notes. Aidan is crying as he is overly tired and Ethan is throwing up—something he does readily whenever he is jostled.

The extent SID will play in our lives won't become evident until two years from now. That's when Aidan will begin his meltdowns of panic attacks when he is in a public place—especially one brimming with too much stimulus like a children's play center.

Makes me wonder; why is it clinics specializing in caring for toddlers with *sensory issues* have waiting rooms filled with too many lights, constant sound from TV monitors, and a jumble of brightly colored decorations?

Chapter 30 - *Fast Forward: One to Five*

"...and thank you for a house full of people I love. Amen."
Ward Elliot Hour

Age – One Year

I have been told numerous times that this journey of recovery from extreme premature birth would take five to seven years before we would know which disabilities would be considered permanent.

For the next five years (or perhaps longer), numerous specialists will monitor my boys and I will continue recording medical updates in my journal.

Let's face it; recovery does not happen magically upon discharge from the NICU, or upon reaching the first birthday. I need to pace my expectations and start thinking of progress in yearly increments.

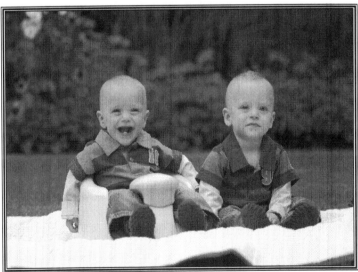

Age 1 yr. - Ethan (in booster seat to sit upright) and Aidan

In this first year, the boys are hospitalized several times with pneumonia. Aidan recovers rapidly after each hospitalization, but Ethan takes much longer as he struggles to breathe. Our house is once again filled with oxygen tanks.

To celebrate the boys' first birthday, we hold a party to honor the miracle of life fought for and won by one-pound babies. Family, friends, NICU nurses, and respiratory therapists attend—even Dr. Lim and Dr. Placket come!

***

Aidan is 16 pounds and crawling with ease. He tries to escape his playpen by standing on a toy to look over the top of the rail—as if surveying his escape route.

He loves peek-a-boo, babbles with an animated voice and has an infectious giggle. Aidan loves to splash in the bath and has a smile that warms your heart. He has no fear and will launch himself towards whatever catches his attention. The dog and cats have learned to steer clear of his reach.

This little guy has an insatiable desire to read books. Fortunately, Nana and Papa oblige him with limitless story time. It is uncanny how his fingers touch each word on the page as if he is checking to be sure no words are skipped.

***

Ethan weighs in at a scant 13 pounds. He is closer to figuring out how to crawl. Has all the motions—just needs to put them together in the right sequence.

This little one's chest muscles are not strong enough to sit upright, so a special booster seat is used for meals. He will tolerate sitting up for a short while, but would rather lie on his activity mat. Ethan smiles, but rarely makes any sound. I am not sure he realizes yet that he has a voice box. Perhaps the ventilator tubes kept him silent for too long.

We are watchful for signs of cerebral palsy and learning difficulties caused by the brain bleed. So far I see no concrete indicators, but I do notice Ethan has the unusual habit of intently inspecting a toy from all angles before he will play with it. It is as if he is mentally dismantling and reassembling the toy piece-by-piece inside his head.

Age – Two Years

Due to the boys' weak immune systems and compromised lungs, we are house-bound. Despite this isolation, both boys continue to end up in the hospital with pneumonia. Even the dreaded RSV finds a way into our house.

My so-called 'social calendar' is limited to multiple trips each week to see the specialists monitoring the boys. But isolation doesn't mean boring! We turned our family room into a giant playpen filled with books and toys to promote both physical and mental growth. Nana and Papa come everyday to help. The boys love the attention and I sure love the extra hands!

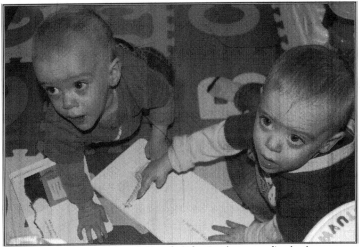

Age Two – Ethan (left) and Aidan in playpen reading books

***

At age 2 yrs. 6 mos., Aidan has his first seizure. He toddles into the family room blabbing happily, then suddenly grows quite and stands eerily still. His expressive eyes go blank into a fixed unseeing stare. Aidan's arms hang limp and his hands flutter at his sides. I try to rouse him but he is unresponsive. This episode lasts for less than a minute but it feels like an hour.

The doc is not sure what may have triggered this. It could very well be nothing more a random symptom from a former-preemie whose brain is still developing.

Over the next several months, Aidan continues to have these mild seizure-like symptoms. We are referred to a neurologist who agrees with a seizure diagnosis. EKGs are ordered to rule out epilepsy.

Keeping Aidan lying perfectly still for the EKG is a test of wills. I cajole and finally bribe him with the promise of a new storybook. Aidan has probes stuck all over his scalp and he counters back in sign language holding up three fingers to indicate he wants *three* new storybooks. Anything baby, anything. Just hold still.

After hours of testing, the results are inconclusive. The seizures are just something we hope he'll outgrow.

***

By age 2 yrs. 9 mos., Aidan develops night terrors. This is *not* a nightmare. I can deal with nightmares. A night terror is altogether a different matter. This is when a toddler has a sudden awakening from a deep sleep with screaming, profuse sweating, confusion, extremely rapid heart rate, and hallucinations.

It doesn't make me feel any better to learn that night terrors are relatively rare—occurring in just 3-to-6% of children and are more typically found in boys.

The doctor tries to reassure me saying most children have only one or two episodes lasting just one to five minutes. He adds that toddlers will spontaneously cease to have night terrors in a few weeks as the nervous system matures.

This update means nothing to me as Aidan's night terrors have been going on now for months—and each episode lasts 50 to 60 minutes!

When Aidan has a night terror, he sits bolt upright and jumps from his bed, flails his arms, and screams non-stop in pure terror. His eyes are wide open but unseeing. He is inconsolable and does not recognize Justin or me. I try to wake him, but this does not work and causes him even more distress.

At the end of a night terror, Aidan will collapse in a heap on the floor and has no memory of this episode. I scoop him up in my arms and put him back to bed.

I find I can stop most night terrors from starting if I catch one in the early stages. When Aidan starts to fuss or cry out in his sleep, I wake him with a gentle touch and hold him in my arms until he falls back to sleep. This means every night I lie on the floor next to Aidan's bed—never totally relaxing, as I keep tuned for a sign that another night terror may be starting.

***

Not all our focus at age two is on health issues. This is also a time of remarkable surprises and great joy.

Looking back over my journal notes I come across an entry made when Ethan is two and a half years old. I wrote:

Ethan said his FIRST WORD!

Except it wasn't exactly a *word*, rather he recited several alphabet letters! This comes as a shock as I did not teach him this.

I need to explain. I expected his first word would be *mama*. During playtime I repeated *mama* over and over to stack the deck as to what the boys' first word would be—but neither boy ever mimicked this sound.

The speech therapist told me not to worry. She comments that boys tend to talk late, and twins tend to talk later still.

So imagine my surprise when Ethan, looking at bright colored alphabet magnets scattered in random order across the refrigerator door, started naming the letters!

How did he learn the alphabet? Was it the bright colored letters on his playpen mat? Was it the hours of reading storybooks, or his alphabet puzzles?

I'll never know. All I know is Ethan's first word was not *mama*, but rather, "p, b, m, n, d, g..." Each letter is vocalized clearly in the same sequence as the corresponding alphabet magnet lined-up on the refrigerator door.

Age – Three years

It has been three years and we still struggle with financial and medical issues. Medical bills since the boys' birth now total more than $2.3 million—and there is no end in sight. Federal aid is available when an earthquake or hurricane knocks down your home. But there is no relief program when the storm is in the form of insurmountable medical bills. The system is set that you must loose everything you have before help is available.

After liquidating Justin's company, we sold our car, emptied our savings and retirement accounts, and leveraged our home equity. We even sold off nearly all our possessions. But the medical bills continued to pile on. In rapid succession we lost our lovely home and filed for bankruptcy. It is all gone.

As devastating as this is, I tell myself this is just a loss of *things*. If I don't take this attitude I will become bitterly depressed. I need to focus on what we do have—our boys, our family, and our love for each other.

***

The medical issues continue to plague Ethan. He has 'failure to thrive' and is not growing. At age three he ends up with the surgically implanted G-tube. He tolerates this procedure quite well, and by the second day after surgery we're giving him and his buddy Elmo rides up and down the Pediatric floor in a wheelchair shaped like a racecar.

I sew Ethan's t-shirts into onesies so his little Houdini-hands can't get at the G-tube to pull it out. If it comes out we're back for more surgery. Ethan will wear these altered tee shirts for several years yet to come.

He'll need the nightly G-tube feedings until just before his fifth birthday. When the tube is finally removed, it will leave a graphic, bullet hole-like scar. I can just imagine the elaborate stories Ethan will make-up to explain this scar!

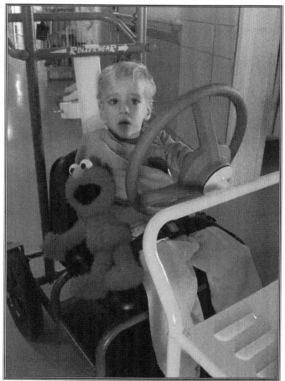

Age Three - Ethan & Elmo cruise the hospital hallways

***

Our evenings follow a repetitive regiment. First is bath time with much laughter and splashing of soapy water. Then comes pajamas and story time while Ethan is hooked up for his nighttime feeding. He has to lie flat on his back so the tubing does not kink and block the flow of formula. If the line is blocked, the monitor on the IV pole sounds an alarm.

This is a slow process. It takes eight hours for the two bags of formula to drip into his stomach. Ever try to keep a three year old lying flat for eight hours? I think I could enter this as a new Olympic event!

I never know which boy will need me during the night. If Aidan wakes from a deep dream state, it will trigger night terrors. So I have to wake him *before* the terrors start. If Ethan rolls over in his sleep (which he does several times a night) the feeding line kinks and sets off the alarm. I gently roll him onto his back and straighten the tubing before the contraption spills the expensive formula all over the bed.

Tending to both boys all night long is so exhausting that I don't even bother to go to bed myself. Most nights it doesn't seem worth the energy to crawl back to own my bedroom. I have my pillow stuffed under Aidan's bed so I can just pull it out and sleep right there on the floor.

***

At age three, neither boy is overly verbal; but there is something unusual going on. While Aidan and Ethan don't speak, *they spell!* Okay, I know this sounds like a wild exaggeration—but they are spelling words.

What words? The easy ones are 'cat' and 'dog'...but the shocker is they spell more readily than speak when asked a question.

I ask Ethan, "What animals begin with the letter D?"

His reply is captured in the photo!

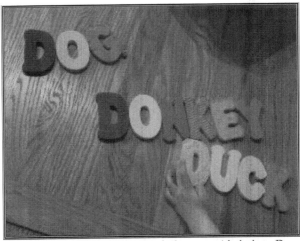

Age Three - Ethan spells animals that start with the letter D

Age – Four years

Shortly before the boys' fourth birthday, we're told their immune systems are now strong enough to leave home isolation. Yahoo! I love my boys, but I am starved for some people-time of my own.

With this good news, I plan my return to work. We need the extra income desperately to get back our financial independence. Returning to work means either daycare or a nanny. Since daycare is the least costly of the two options, that's what we chose.

I was warned daycare would expose the boys to many viruses. Sure enough, both caught a series of colds that land them back in the hospital with pneumonia. Daycare is a short-lived option. After several months attempting to make this work, we decide what we really need is a nanny.

Selecting a nanny was easy this time. The twins' beloved teacher from daycare, Miss Rachel, agrees to care for the boys. It's a perfect choice, as they adore her. Ethan even wrote a story for Miss Rachel that he fashioned into a maze.

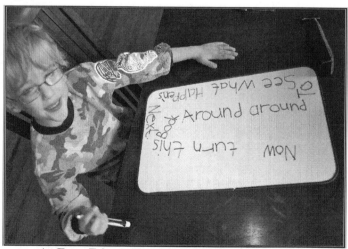

Age Four - Ethan writes a story he titles "The Maze of Words"

More good news—by age four Aidan's nervous system matures and his seizures and night terrors stop. It was like a switch was turned off. We went from having several episodes a month to none. They stopped suddenly—just as Dr. Clausen predicted they would.

***

We are off to the neurologist for a routine exam. This appointment is part of the monitoring to check for problems in brain development due to the boys' extreme prematurity and brain hemorrhage.

As the doctor enters the room, Aidan hides under my coat—so the examination starts first with Ethan.

The neurologist has a series of questions for me.

"Does Ethan talk?" *No, neither boy talks much yet.*

"Does Ethan dress himself?" *No, the feeding tube protruding from his belly makes getting dressed difficult.*

"Does Ethan run, jump, or climb?" *Not much. He tires so easily that he prefers to ride in a wagon to walking or running.*

"Does Ethan recognize any alphabet letters?"

Okay, how to answer this last question stops me cold.

I tell the doctor that both boys know their alphabet letters and they can spell words.

The neurologist turns to Ethan and says, "My, oh my, Ethan. So you can spell! Can you spell CAT?"

Ethan looks up from his iPod with a bored expression and shakes his head. Then he returns his attention to his hand-held computer word game.

I know Ethan won't cooperate to spell easy words. He needs a challenge; so I say to the doctor, "Ask him to spell something harder—like a three syllable word."

The doctor is probably thinking this is a ridiculous game and wants to end it before it gets out of hand. Picking a three-syllable word out of the air, he says to Ethan, "Ok son. Can you spell ADVENTURE?"

Ethan grins mischievously, and then looks up to the right as if he can see the letters assemble themselves in mid air. After a pause of 10 seconds he enunciates each letter clearly saying, "A D V E N T U R..."

Pausing for dramatic effect before saying the last letter, Ethan says "B". Then he laughs and quickly adds, "No, not **B**...it's **E** for Ethan!" He smiles at his own joke of intentionally inserting the wrong letter at the end of the word.

The doctor drops his pen onto his lap and it rolls onto the floor. He sits for several seconds just staring at Ethan.

Breaking into a wide grin he says, "There's nothing wrong with this kid's brain!"

***

Speaking in sentences came late for my boys, but as if by magic shortly after their fourth birthday they burst into non-stop talking. Clarity of their words is still an issue, but weekly speech therapy is helping.

When they are not talking, they are writing full sentences and practice different fonts (yes, Ethan has moved on from simple upper and lower case letters to experimenting with serif and sans serif fonts).

Ethan loves to write stories and his meticulously precise handwriting fills every scrape of paper in the house.

I ran out of paper once and that was a disaster. Ethan was in the midst of writing a story and there was not enough paper left to finish his project. He decides to take measures into his own hands and continues writing his story in black felt pen across the wall. What a sight. Justin has to repaint the entire living room wall to cover up Ethan's handiwork.

***

While Ethan is the writer, Aidan is the avid reader and imaginative storyteller. If Aidan is not reading, he is playing computer strategy games.

I overheard Aidan reading aloud from a new storybook he picked out just this morning at the library. It is about a class of children visiting a reptile zoo. In his animated storyteller voice Aidan reads aloud, "...and then the anaconda slithered out of the pond..."

Now, I can see how he could sound out the word 'anaconda' but where the heck did he learn how to pronounce the word 'slithered'?

He finishes his library book and climbs up on the kitchen stool to use my laptop. Aidan switches the computer on and opens a math strategy game. After advancing a few levels, he says he is stuck and needs help.

Glancing at the screen, I readily see I have absolutely no idea how to solve this strategy puzzle. I suggest, "Why don't you just move on to another game?"

Aidan gives me an exasperated look as if to say, *Quit the game? No way!* He considers the puzzle a bit longer and figures out a solution.

"Look Mommy," he says, "this is how you do it!"

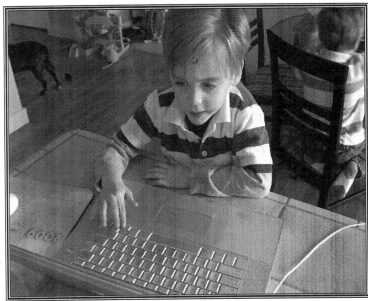

Age Four - Aidan working computer strategy games

Age – Five Years

The fifth year, like all the prior years, brings a full battery of tests by a long list of specialists who have monitored the twins since birth. We've spent time with a pediatric heart specialist for aortic root dilatation; gastroenterologist for feeding and growth; pulmonologist for lungs severely scarred; neurologist for brain bleeds and seizures; ophthalmologist for vision issues; and speech and physical therapists for muscles that lack coordination.

Today is a very important appointment with our wonderful primary care pediatrician, Dr. Clausen. This is the fifth year checkup and I am anxious to hear which of the health issues are considered resolved and which are likely to remain.

As Dr. Clausen enters the exam room he has a chipper voice and says, "Hello boys! Who wants to be the first one examined?"

Aidan doesn't miss a beat. Without looking up from his handheld computer he deadpans, "Ethan will go first."

Ethan looks like a deer caught in headlights. He can't think of anything fast enough to put the attention back onto his brother. Lacking any delay tactics, Ethan is hoisted up onto the exam table.

After each boy is done with their physical exam, it is time for their vaccinations. Dr. Clausen says, "Okay boys. Just a quick poke and we'll be all done."

Two nurses assist to get this over with fast before either boy realizes what is in store. Their middle finger is pricked for the blood test and then five vaccinations in the thigh for each boy. All of course, received with tears and loud protests.

The exam room has a chalkboard placed at a kid-friendly height. Ethan promptly climbs down from the exam table and picking up a piece of chalk writes a message on the board for Dr. Clausen—complete with punctuation and quotation marks.

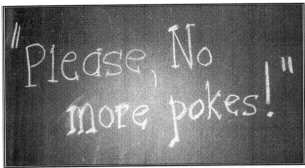

Ethan writes a message for Dr. Clausen

Tapping the chalk against the board with one hand and pointing at Dr. Clausen, Ethan says with all the seriousness he can muster; "Doctor, can you read this please?"

Ethan's antics break everyone up. As the nurses laugh and prepare to leave the exam room, Aidan wipes tears from his face. He says with a teary voice, "That was not *one poke*. That was six pokes for me and six pokes for Ethan. That is twelve many pokes!"

Dr. Clausen sits staring incredulously.

He finally speaks. "I think you have remarkably gifted boys. I have seen only one other child in my career come even close to this...but your two just blow me away. I think you're in for a wild time keeping them challenged."

***

Dr. Clausen shifts in his chair as he reaches for the twins' hefty medical charts.

This is it! The update I have been waiting five years to hear comes next. I will finally learn which health issues will shadow the boys' future.

Since the beginning, all I ever wanted to know was *will my sons survive?* And if so, *will they have disabilities?*

My boys have battled so many dragons on their journey through the world of extreme prematurity; but in this moment it comes to me—if any dragons remain, the boys will tame them to be a quiet presence in their lives.

I lay my pen down. There is nothing more to write.

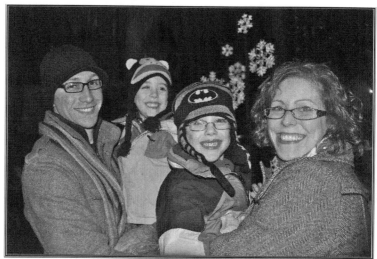

Daddy and Aidan, Ethan and Mommy
December 2011

While this is the last chapter of the twins' five-year journal, their story does not have an ending—only a beginning. The rest of the story is for the twins to tell. And I am sure my boys will have delightful stories filled with love, challenges, and achievements.

The boys think every day is made just for them. They marvel at ordinary things—a leaf, a storybook, a rain puddle. They chase butterflies, collect twigs, and stuff ants in their pockets.

They amaze me.

Bath time is chaos of splashing.

Story time trumps all playtime.

They give out kisses and hugs.

And they are loved.

Research for Prevention of Preterm Birth

The prevalence of preterm birth and stillbirth constitutes a global health crisis resulting in millions of maternal and newborn deaths every year. It brings untold economic and social costs. Babies who survive preterm birth may suffer life-long consequences, including cerebral palsy, vision loss, learning difficulties, chronic lung disease, hearing loss, and autism.

Can we help more babies to survive prematurity? Can we find a way to prevent preterm and stillbirths some day? In the 1960's, a premature baby born at 28 weeks almost never survived. With research, by the time the 1980's came around, babies born at 28 weeks had a 20% chance of survival. Now in 2011, babies at 28 weeks have a 90% survival rate.[26] And survival rates for babies born before 28 weeks gestation are also on the rise.

Premature baby survival rates are one way to measure success. However, the most meaningful measurement will be found in the number of preterm births prevented.

Preventing pre-term births, and developing successful solutions to treat premature babies, requires research and funding.

March of Dimes

In 2005, the March of Dimes began the Prematurity Research Initiative (PRI), which funds innovative research into the causes of prematurity. More than $15 million has been awarded to 43 grantees over the past six years. Some PRI grantees are exploring how genetics or a combination of genetic and environmental factors may influence a

---

[26] Centers for Disease Control and Prevention, August 2011, www.cdc.gov.

woman's chances of going into labor prematurely. Others are examining how infections may trigger early labor. One of every three premature births can be attributed to an infection in a woman's uterus, which may have had no warning symptoms.

In addition to PRI support, the March of Dimes funds national prematurity research programs. Grantees are improving the care of premature babies by developing new ways to help prevent or treat common complications of prematurity. For example, researchers helped develop surfactant treatment, which has saved tens of thousands of premature babies with breathing problems.

To bring this issue to the attention of the media, March of Dimes[27] sponsors *World Prematurity Day* each year on November 17th to honor the million babies worldwide who died that year simply because they were born too soon, and to honor the 12 million more who struggle to survive their premature birth.

GAAPS

GAPPS (Global Alliance to Prevent Prematurity and Stillbirth)[28], funded by the Bill and Melinda Gates Foundation, is spearheading one of the largest ever international research efforts focused exclusively on pregnancy. Experts from around the world are teaming up in studies that may some day solve preterm birth—and along the way develop effective treatment interventions.

This research is targeted on understanding the genetics and biology of a normal pregnancy. Studies on a normal pregnancy have been rather limited to date, creating a huge deficit in our knowledge of the causes of stillbirth and prematurity. This knowledge gap is one of the greatest

---

[27] Dr. Jennifer Howse, President, March of Dimes, Jun 2010, marchofdimes.com.

[28] Dr. Craig Rubens, Executive Director, GAPPS, Nov 2011, GAPPSSeattle.org.

barriers to developing effective diagnostic, prevention and treatment interventions. With this data, researchers can conduct studies that could lead to life-saving prevention techniques and therapies for preterm birth.

GAAPS convened medical experts from around the world at their 2009 International Conference on Prematurity and Stillbirth to launch initiatives to find creative solutions to improve maternal, fetal, newborn and child health. These complex problems require an interdisciplinary research approach and an international commitment.

***

As a young child in the 1950's, my mom recalls going door-to-door with her mother to collect coins for the March of Dimes to solve the crisis of polio. Research successfully solved polio within my mother's lifetime. Now researchers are tackling preterm birth and I am hopeful they will solve the crisis of prematurity during my lifetime—or certainly within the lifetime of my sons.

Mom (aka Nana) is now retired and serves as a volunteer lobbyist for premature birth research; and I am a member of the Tiny Footprints Guild—dedicated to raising awareness and funding for research initiatives sponsored Seattle Children's Hospital to champion those born with 'tiny footprints'.

You can learn more about research efforts to solve preterm birth by visiting the web sites for GAPPS.org and MarchofDimes.com.

Discussion Questions

Q. Your family was bankrupted by your babies' premature birth. What words would you pass on to those trying to address a federal healthcare program?

There must be an annual cap on out-of-pocket expenses for each family. The health care reform introduced back in 2010 has gaps. One gap is the lack of a cap on the maximum a family will pay for medical bills.

There is federal help if a hurricane wipes out your home, but there is no help if medical bills erase your entire net worth. I believe a system could be employed to cover catastrophic events through private insurance pools just as the government covers certificates of deposit.

Choosing between financial stability and the life of your child should never be a choice forced on any family.

Q. The divorce rate for families dealing with critically ill or disabled children is as high as 80%. Did this experience impact your marriage?

Every aspect of my life was upside down—my children were critically ill, we lost our home, our savings and retirement accounts were wiped out, my husband lost his company, and my career evaporated. About the only thing that did survive intact was my marriage.

I saw other NICU families falter and marriages break under the strain. The impact of constant stress of a critically ill child and medical debt can be an unrelenting burden on marriage.

The divorce rate in families with critically ill or disabled children is astronomical. If healthcare reforms place a cap on families' out-of-pocket medical costs, it may end up saving more than just money.

Q. What advice would you give to a medical team on how to talk with the parent of a preemie?

The NICU teams are dealing with parents at an extremely emotional time. Communication needs to be frequent and often repeated. It needs to be empathetic, realistic, and delivered with care so the light of hope survives.

Don't take it personally if I ask you to explain your opinion or if I challenge a course of action that you recommend. I am struggling with overwhelming emotions and I may need to hear your points over and over again before I can comprehend what you are trying to tell me.

Be honest, but don't focus just on the worst-case statistics. Take the time to share all the possible outcomes and options, and let me take a moment to process this.

Q. How would you recommend parents talk with the medical team?

Insist the doctor give an understandable explanation of their medical opinion. If you don't understand what is said, ask the doctor to repeat it—or ask the doctor to draw a picture if necessary.

Be considerate of the doctors' time and come prepared with a list of your questions. Take notes and write down the doctor's counsel and answers to your questions.

It can be hard to listen when you're under the stress of a critically ill baby; so taking notes is a good way to focus your hearing and to keep on task with your questions. And be sure to ask for the correct spelling so you can do a little research yourself on the Internet.

Not all Internet sites are reliable. Some sites are better than others. Web sites maintained by children's hospitals, American Academy of Pediatrics, American Academy of Family Physicians, or the March of Dimes are examples of the more reliable sites.

Q. What advice would you pass on to NICU parents?

Be an advocate for your baby. The NICU environment can be intimidating. You need to be the one who speaks up for your baby. You are their champion who looks out for their best interest. You are the most important thing in your baby's life.

Join a parents group. Talk to other NICU parents and learn from them how to navigate your own journey. If there isn't a group at your NICU, ask to join one at a nearby hospital. Or join one online. Enter key words (such as NICU Parent Group, or Preemie Parent Group) into an Internet search engine and you'll find listings of group sites.

Keep a journal. There is so much information thrown at you, it may be impossible to process it all. Keeping a journal will help you track your child's progress and allow you to have some level of control in what is often an out-of-control situation.

Insist on financial counseling from the very start. In the first days of the NICU ask your hospital to assign a Medical Social Worker with the skills to help you navigate financial issues. Also, ask the hospital to predict the total hospitalization bill, and ask your pediatrician and other healthcare providers to estimate post-discharge expenses for the next two to three years. Armed with this information seek counsel from an attorney, financial planner, or other professional on options available to meet this anticipated medical debt. With constant changes in insurance policies and federal programs, you'll need a plan to navigate the financial side of a preterm baby.

We would love to hear from you.
You can email the authors at

apoundofhope@me.com

Michele Kemper
(aka Nana)

Jen Sinconis
(aka Mama)

Made in the USA
Lexington, KY
23 August 2012